Praise for Crunch a Color and *The 52 New Foods Challenge*

"Fun? Simple? Rewards dinner conversation, good manners,
and setting the table? Encourages even the most reticent child—or adult!—
to eat their veggies? Supports nonprofits dedicated to combating the
childhood obesity epidemic? You can see why we love this game."

—LAURIE DAVID'S *The Family Dinner*

"A simple, fun, and playful way to get kids to eat healthy and try new foods."

—RACHAEL RAY'S *Yum-o!*

"A mom and genius game creator helping kids eat fresh food!"

—JAMIE OLIVER'S *Food Revolution*

"Invites kids of all ages into the kitchen to cook, and gives them exactly what they need to
get excited about kale, salmon, and quinoa instead of pasta, pizza, and other 'kid food.'
Jennifer Tyler Lee has planted the seeds of comfort and confidence in the child's kitchen."

—JESSE COOL, AUTHOR OF *Simply Organic*

"A year from reading this book, the fact that your family is eating healthier will be a symptom
of something far deeper. The food will have been a delicious prop, an opportunity to think
and communicate differently. That's what makes Jennifer Tyler Lee's book so valuable. If it
helps, think of *The 52 New Foods Challenge* as a delicious blend of Dr. Spock and *The Joy of
Cooking* for twenty-first-century foodie parents. But it's much more than that."

—RAJ PATEL, AUTHOR OF *Stuffed and Starved*

The 52 New Foods Challenge

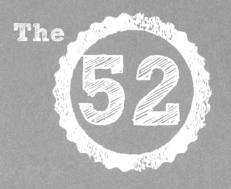

The 52 NEW FOODS CHALLENGE

A Family Cooking Adventure for Each Week of the Year

WITHDRAWN

Jennifer Tyler Lee

AVERY

a member of Penguin Group (USA)

New York

Published by the Penguin Group
Penguin Group (USA) LLC
375 Hudson Street
New York, New York 10014

USA • Canada • UK • Ireland • Australia
New Zealand • India • South Africa • China

penguin.com
A Penguin Random House Company

Most Avery books are available at special quantity discounts for bulk purchase for sales promotions, premiums,
fund-raising, and educational needs. Special books or book excerpts also can be created to fit specific needs.
For details, write Special.Markets@us.penguingroup.com.

Library of Congress Cataloging-in-Publication Data

Lee, Jennifer Tyler.
The 52 new foods challenge : a family cooking adventure for each week of the year / Jennifer Tyler Lee.
        p.   cm.
Includes index.
ISBN 978-1-58333-556-7
1. Seasonal cooking.   2. Families—Nutrition.   3. Food habits.   4. Adventure games.
I. Title.   II. Title: Fifty-two new foods challenge.
TX714.L4426   2014   2014027128
641.5′64—dc23

Printed in the United States of America
1   3   5   7   9   10   8   6   4   2

BOOK DESIGN BY TANYA MAIBORODA

For Catherine, James, and Anthony,

who fill me up

with love

Contents

Summer

Foreword

GETTING KIDS TO EAT HEALTHY FOOD IS THE GREATEST CHALLENGE WE FACE—NOT ONLY AS parents but also as a nation. We live in an era when our children's life spans may be shorter than those of their parents', an era when cancer is the foremost cause of death of children under fifteen, an era when diabetes and obesity are rampant—three times the rate of a generation ago. It will take us all to reverse these stats.

And it will take healthy, unprocessed food.

Food literacy must be one of our most important goals in overcoming our country's food and health crises. But where do we start? It begins by finding our kitchens again; and not only finding them but also sharing them with our families—and most especially our kids! Schools can be part of the solution, but parents also have a major role to play.

Enter *The 52 New Foods Challenge* by Jennifer Tyler Lee.

In this book, and the Crunch a Color game that complements it, we meet a mom, advocate, and inspiration who helps families move from bland to bountiful plates—from the freezer section to the farmers' market. Through an ingenious and simple game, *The 52 New Foods Challenge* inspires kids, their parents, friends, and families to get into the kitchen to cook, taste, and eat healthy, unprocessed foods—together.

I believe that the 52 New Foods Challenge is a positive journey that every family can embark on. With it we can truly change not only our children's relationship with food but also our own. This book may actually help families save the health of our children, our nation, and perhaps our planet as well!

—Chef Ann Cooper

A Note to the Reader

THE 52 NEW FOODS CHALLENGE IS ABOUT MORE THAN THE FOODS—IT'S ABOUT THE JOURNEY the foods take you on. Along the way, you will experience failures and frustrations, successes and celebrations. In the end, though, you will transform the way your family eats because of the experience you have together.

Maybe your kids refuse to eat their vegetables and you're at your breaking point. Or you feel like you've done everything right, preparing wholesome meals from the start, and all of a sudden your kids no longer eat the healthy foods they once did. You may have a family that eats healthy most of the time, but you're looking for ways to break your recipe rut and try something new. Regardless of the reason, the solution lies in taking the journey together.

I started the 52 New Foods Challenge to get my kids past pasta and peas and to encourage them to be more willing to try new foods. What I discovered was that the journey wasn't about getting my kids to change. It was about creating a change in me. The 52 New Foods Challenge transformed me, which in turn transformed our family dinners.

The key to making a change at your family table lies in learning to see things in a new light—to change your perspective. That's hard. This book will help you get there. Peppered throughout this book, I have included stories from my family's adventure—what worked and what didn't—and practical tips to help you achieve your goal. My hope is that my story will inspire your story. Meet your family where they are, and move forward from there. Everyone will start at a different place, and everyone can make lasting changes. This is your family's adventure, and like any good recipe, the secret is to make it your own.

—Jennifer

The 52 New Foods Challenge

Introduction

In every job that must be done
There is an element of fun
You find the fun, and snap!
The job's a game.
—MARY POPPINS

Where We Began

When my daughter, Catherine, was two, she ate everything. A happy little sprout, she would bounce around the table snatching and sampling healthy bits of food until her big, round belly was satisfied. I was a beaming mom. To be sure, she had her go-to favorites like "habas" (otherwise known as strawberries) and "mum mums" (her code for mushrooms), but for the most part she had a pretty broad palate and was willing to try new foods without much fuss. Naively, I thought I had avoided picky-eater syndrome and the terrible dinner struggles that plagued most of my friends at the time.

But as we inched toward kindergarten, my proud-parent glow faded as my daughter's interest in a colorful plate waned. How could it be that yesterday she loved broccoli and today she ran from it as if it were a dragon with fangs? Instead of a colorful rainbow of healthy, wholesome foods, her plate looked more like a tired ski run at the end of a long winter season—whitish brown with a few trampled sprigs of green peeking out here and there, longing for a taste of spring sunshine. Even worse, my diet seemed to be trailing downhill along with hers. "Why bother to cook it if she's not going to eat it?" I reasoned, as my healthy diet was reduced to pasta and peas. Dinner was dreary.

"Don't give her an option!"

"Picky eaters are made, not born!"

"One family, one meal."

"If she doesn't eat what you serve, she'll be hungry and eat at the next meal."

This was the advice I got from trusted doctors and family friends, but I was completely unwilling to swallow it. Forcing my kids to eat went against every single motherly instinct in my body. To me, it felt like a military deployment: Make a plan, send out your best troops, and stick to your guns with an unrelenting will to wear the enemy down. I didn't want mealtime to become a battleground in my family.

I tried to understand why Catherine was becoming pickier, but her fickleness made no sense to me. "What child doesn't like bananas?" I would ask rhetorically. I was immensely frustrated. All of that frustration spilled over onto the dinner table, and though I'd vowed not to let it happen, mealtime became an experience that we all wanted to avoid. I bargained and bribed. I begged and badgered. At my lowest point, I heard myself screaming, "Why won't you eat your vegetables?" What I hadn't realized was that I was asking the wrong question.

I needed to be asking myself, "Why *will* my kids eat their vegetables?" It's a subtle difference, but that change invited a playful challenge to be taken on together as opposed to setting up a challenge against me.

I was desperate for a solution and equally determined not to give up. I wanted the dinner table to be a place where we gathered for wholesome food, good fun, and treasured time together. I knew there was a better way, I just didn't know how to get there—yet.

A surprise moment during a typical Monday morning routine gave me the inspiration. My husband, Anthony, was getting the kids washed, brushed, dressed, and ready for school. On the days when I was in charge of getting everyone out the door, there was usually rushing and barking involved (and I'm not talking about our family dog). But Anthony has a magical way of making just about anything fun. That morning, after they worked on a Lego project in the living room, he started to get the kids ready for school. "Race ya!" he yelled as he charged up the stairs to brush his teeth. "Let's see if we can beat our record getting to school this morning!" he challenged. Giggling and skipping, my kids happily got themselves organized and were out the door, backpacks and lunches in tow, without any screaming or cajoling required. I watched the whole thing unfold as if I were watching a movie—with awe and disbelief. As the car door slammed and they cruised down the street, an idea popped into my head: "Why don't I make healthy eating a game?"

Making It a Game

That night, I made up a dinner game based on earning points by eating different colors. The premise was simple—more colorful vegetables and fruits meant a healthier meal. The more challenging the food, the more points you could earn: 5 for apples, 10 for broccoli, and 15 for kale. Bonus points for trying a new food.

Kale becomes cool when it's worth 15 points, and the race for bonus points suddenly had my kids begging for new foods to try. Beans, broccoli, and even Brussels sprouts started showing up regularly at our family dinners. Not every food was met with a joyously warm welcome, but we were heading down the right path. With care and time, our simple mealtime game grew organically around our family table, rooting its way into the fabric of our meals, until counting colors became second nature. When a nutritionist I met with said, "This is exactly how we teach about nutrition, but it's way more fun!" I realized that I might be onto something.

My kids embraced the idea and helped me to create Crunch a Color, an award-winning healthy-eating game that is now sold nationwide. Suddenly, my in-box was filled with messages from parents around the country sharing stories about how this simple game was changing the way their kids looked at vegetables—as a fun challenge rather than a forced mandate. Making healthy eating a game not only worked at our table, it was also working at tables across the country.

52 New Foods

In my family, Crunch a Color was the start of our new, healthier relationship with food. It got us out of an intractable place. It made food fun and reduced stress at our family table. More important, making healthy eating a game opened the door to even bigger changes for our family, the kind that would establish a lifetime of healthy eating habits—for all of us.

My kids were now counting their colors without much prompting from me. They knew what a balanced plate looked like. Their favorite part of the game was to earn a card that would double all of their points by trying something new. That simple challenge helped pique a willingness to try new foods. So at the beginning of the new year, we decided to take on a family challenge: 52 weeks, 52 new foods.

I knew that for any change to stick, it had to be simple. Saying that we were going to "eat healthy" was too broad (and overwhelming). On the other hand, saying we were going to try one new food each week, and cook it together as a family, felt tangible. I knew what that meant, and so did my kids. It also felt like something I could handle—once a week was doable, but anything more felt like way too much for our busy lives. I certainly couldn't commit to cooking at home every night of the week, or going cold turkey on things like canned soups and packaged granola bars, but making a commitment to cook together with my kids once a week felt manageable. We all agreed that this was something fun for us to do as a family. Taking on this challenge together was another essential ingredient to success—that way everyone was working toward the same goal.

Each week, we would head to the farmers' market or local grocery store, and my kids would choose a new, healthy food to try. Like players in a scavenger hunt, my new-food adventurers would race from stall to stall, scouting out our new food of the week. Sometimes it was a vegetable that we had yet to try together, like artichoke or zucchini. Other times it was a seasonal favorite that we decided to try in a new way, like cherries or plums. This simple activity kept us focused on local, seasonal produce (and away from anything that arrived in a box, bag, or can). Then together, we would cook. "Easy enough for a five-year-old to make!" was our mantra. Cooking together as a family, we learned to make easy, healthy recipes that we could all enjoy. We chronicled the entire journey, keeping track of favorite ingredients, quick tips, and easy recipes, making it simple to stay on track. Unusual new foods like Romanesco and quinoa joined us for dinner, along with familiar favorites prepared in new ways. But the change to healthier eating wasn't because I was dictating the menu with a tiger mom's iron fist. Our 52 New Foods Challenge worked because it was easy and fun for the whole family—it engaged all of us.

At the time I thought this challenge would simply be a way to get my kids to try a few new foods—to add variety to our table beyond broccoli, beans, and blueberries. What I discovered was that the 52 New Foods Challenge was the catalyst for much deeper and longer-lasting changes in the way that we were eating—not just for my kids but for our whole family. The 52 New Foods Challenge laid the foundation for a lifetime of positive and healthy eating habits centered on whole, nutritious foods. It brought us together to cook and enjoy healthy food as a family.

Small steps. Big changes.

If I had tried to make all of the changes in this book in one fell swoop, I would have failed. My kids would have thrown up their arms in protest and outright refused to make the changes we needed to make. I can hear it now: "I don't like brown rice!" or "Those vegetables taste too bitter!" or the crowning glory of all comments, "Ew! What's that green stuff?" What's more, I never would have been able to *sustain* the changes—in the way that I shopped, or cooked, or engaged my kids in the whole process. It's the same reason why most diet plans fail—they are impossible to maintain for most people because they don't effect a true change in your lifestyle. The best way to make healthy changes is with small, simple steps taken consistently each week.

The bad news: There isn't a quick fix. Your kids won't go from eating pizza and chicken nuggets to pesto and quinoa in a month, or even three months.

The good news: This plan will work because it changes your family's behavior the slow and sustainable way. The 52 New Foods Challenge helps you make a change at the core of how your family approaches food. You will establish a lifetime of healthy habits by learning to explore and enjoy healthy foods together as a family. And establishing healthy habits at an early age has a dramatic, positive impact on the health of your child throughout his or her life. As noted by Dr. Walter Willett, the head of nutrition at Harvard University's School of Public Health, "This has a direct effect because we have seen diets of children being related to risks of cancer and other conditions later in life."

And it takes only an hour each week, so that even the busiest of parents can help their families make positive changes that will stick.

It was the small steps we took together each week that resulted in a change that could really take hold in our family. It allowed healthy habits to sink in and take root. It took time for me to learn how to cook *with* my kids (not *for* my kids), and for my kids to learn how to cook! Allowing time to explore new foods gave us the opportunity to try lots of different recipes, to experiment with different textures and tastes, and to uncover each person's preferences as opposed to forcing a "one size fits all" approach to food. Just like eating our colors, these healthy habits became second nature because we stuck with them for the long haul. It was the culmination of a series of small steps that resulted in the big, lasting change for our family.

The 52 New Foods Challenge inspired everyone in our family to try something new each week, it encouraged us to start a garden, it brought us together to cook and enjoy healthy food as a family, and it connected us with fellow food lovers in our community. We learned about where our food comes from, the people who work tirelessly to grow it, and how the food choices we make impact our bodies, our neighborhood, and the bigger world around us. We gathered treasured recipes and tips from local farmers, chefs, friends, and family, and together we planted, picked, cooked, and tasted our way through the year. Most important, the 52 New Foods Challenge planted the seeds of change at our family table.

It has the power to seed change at your table, too.

PART 1

Your New Foods Plan

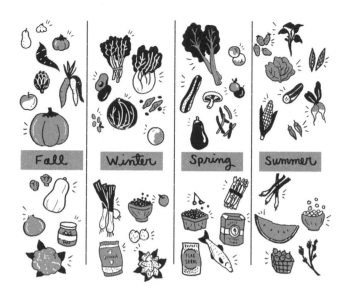

Start Your Challenge

It is better to take many small steps in the right direction
than to make a great leap forward only to stumble backward.
—AN OLD CHINESE PROVERB

YOUR GOAL IS TO TRY ONE NEW FOOD EACH WEEK FOR A YEAR. SMALL STEPS TAKEN CONSIS-
tently will get you there. Remember that the keys to creating a deep and lasting change in
the way that your family eats are to take it slow and to be consistent.

This challenge can feel overwhelming if you don't break it down into manageable parts.
The seasons offer a natural cadence to your 52 New Foods Challenge, making them a great
framework in which to set your goals. Start by committing to try one season's worth of foods.
That's just thirteen weeks—a baker's dozen. Don't worry about how you're going to tackle all
52 weeks. When we started our 52 New Foods Challenge, I remember thinking at week nine,
"How are we going to get through this?" Take it week by week, one season at a time. Each
week I offer a simple activity to work on and easy recipes to try, to keep you moving forward

and having fun. When you complete your first thirteen foods, celebrate your milestone. Use the momentum from the first season to roll into the next.

Where to Begin

The 52 foods are grouped by season so it's easy for you and your family to choose one each week that works best for you and is easily accessible at the market or in your garden. You may already enjoy some of the foods on the list, and that's okay. The point is for you to be cooking together as a family, and a few familiar foods are offered as a bridge to help you get there. Healthy grains and proteins are also offered to help round out your meals.

You can dive right into *The 52 New Foods Challenge* by starting with the season you're in when you opened this book. Commit to trying thirteen new foods together.

52 New Foods

FALL	WINTER	SPRING	SUMMER
1. Sweet Potatoes	14. Kale	27. Asparagus	40. Basil
2. Garlic	15. Radicchio	28. Zucchini	41. Butter Lettuce
3. Artichokes	16. Bok Choy	29. Eggplant	42. Cucumbers
4. Brussels Sprouts	17. Romanesco	30. Green Beans	43. Green Onions
5. Cauliflower	18. Edamame	31. Portobello Mushrooms	44. Radishes
6. Rainbow Carrots	19. Leeks	32. Peas	45. Cherry Tomatoes
7. Pumpkin	20. Avocados	33. Blueberries	46. Corn
8. Butternut Squash	21. Satsuma Mandarin Oranges	34. Strawberries	47. Okra
9. Apples	22. Grapefruits	35. Plums	48. Peaches
10. Pears	23. Kumquats	36. Cherries	49. Watermelon
11. Persimmons	24. Asian Pears	37. Rhubarb	50. Lavender
12. Pomegranates	25. Quinoa	38. Sunflower Butter	51. Flaxseeds
13. Whole Wheat Flour	26. Black Beans	39. Salmon	52. Chickpeas

Many of the recipes in this book are side dishes. That's intentional. It is a risky move to cook a main dish featuring a food that your child has been reluctant to try, only to have them outright refuse to taste it. At that point you're left with one of three options: short-order cook, eat bread, or eat nothing. None of these is a good outcome. There is important learning in the simple act of cooking food together, which I discuss in the Cook Together chapter (page 27), but your long-term success will be built from the momentum that comes from a combination of cooking together and experiencing a series of small successes tasting and trying new foods. Introducing a new food as a side dish, alongside a few favorite foods, is much less daunting than serving it front and center as a main dish. Pair your new foods with a healthy main dish that you know your kids will eat. I've included our family favorites in Appendix A at the back of this book (page 281). I call them Workhorse Recipes, because although they may not be fancy, they are simple, tasty, healthy dishes that I know my kids will eat without a fuss.

Make a Plan and Stick to It

Pick one day each week and make it your New Food Day. Then stick to it. It's easier to make a decision once than to make a decision fifty-two times. Sundays worked best for my family. Choose a day that works best for you. Build in time to shop and chop together, which probably means about two hours each week. The recipes in this book are easy, so they don't require much time, but you'll be more relaxed (and have more fun) if you set aside a few dedicated hours each week with your kids. When you are strapped for time, select the food you plan to try together and do the shopping in advance. Cut the schedule down to *one hour*

Your New Food Day is a great time to prepare a few vegetables for the week ahead. Invite your kids to tear and wash the kale, peel the carrots, and pack veggies in glass containers to make them easy to grab on busy weekdays when time is tight. Whip up a batch of brown rice and keep it the fridge for mixing into dishes all week long. A little prep will go a long way.

each week and use it to cook together. In addition to cooking together as a family on your New Food Day, work your new ingredient into a few of your meals over the course of a month. Prepare your new food two to three different ways, so your kids don't get bored and you can experiment with different tastes and textures. It's important for a new food to show up at your table several times, prepared in several ways—not just one and done. The recipes in this book provide that kind of variety. Your kids might not like radicchio in a salad, but they might like it roasted. You won't know until you try it a few different ways.

Whether you keep a journal, take photos on your phone, or post updates online, record what you learn each week. For my family, keeping a journal in the form of an online blog was the single most important tool for keeping us on target. Your journal, analog or digital, is an easy way to keep you and your family accountable. Jot down tips, favorite ingredients, new foods you would like to try, and simple recipe variations. Snap photos of new foods you discover at the market, candid moments of your family cooking together, and pictures of the meals you create. Let your kids add their notes and musings. Record what is working, along with what isn't. At the end of the year, you will have a treasured family cookbook of healthy foods to enjoy together.

Join the Community

My blog offers a place where you can share your experience with other parents. It's a great way to get the encouragement you'll need to keep going when you hit the tough spots, or to celebrate an accomplishment. It's also packed with tips and tricks. Join me online at www.52newfoods.com.

Keep Score: The Points System

"I hit an all-time high tonight!" James shouted like a gambler on a winning streak. "Over 300 points!" he chuffed to the players at the table, then qualified his winnings with, "I earned a lot of bonus cards this round." He pranced over to the score sheet posted on our fridge to record his accomplishment. New family record.

In this situation, you might think we were talking about a high score in a round of Wii Sports Resort. Or maybe points earned in an old-fashioned game of Scrabble. You might hear boasting in either of those cases, but the win James was talking about was earned for something much different: eating colors.

There are countless systems for teaching families about how to eat healthy. As a child I learned about the food pyramid (yawn), and as a parent I closely watched the renovation of that pyramid into a plate. But for my kids—and me, too those systems are theoretical. They are not engaging. Kids learn through play—interacting with people and the world around them—not through textbooks or food pyramid posters.

Points tap into a child's innate love of games, so they'll get you out of the starting gate. Broccoli is just a stinky green vegetable hogging space on your plate until it's worth 10 points. The points are arbitrary (except that more nutrient-dense and exotic foods are worth more), but points feed our deep-seated drive to make us want to earn them. Use the points system at the beginning of your 52 New Foods Challenge to get you rolling. Know that you will out grow the need for them as your kids learn what a healthy plate looks like.

Track points once a week, on your New Food Day (see page 289 for points by food and how to calculate your score). Use them when you feature your new food on the menu. Dinner worked best for my family, but it could easily be lunch or breakfast. Choose a time that works best for you. At your meal, aim for at least 30 points composed of three colors, one protein, one healthy grain, and one liquid. Points are earned for eating one portion of food: a serving the size of your fist. The smaller the player, the smaller the serving size. Earn as many points for colors (fruits and vegetables) as you like, but limit points for proteins and grains to one serving per meal. Points are also awarded for water and milk, but not juice or soda— removing sugary beverages from your home is one of the simplest changes you can make to help improve the health of your family. Double all of your points if you try something new— even a taster. You can count a food as "new" up to fifteen times. Research shows that it takes

Gateway Foods

For many kids, including my own, branching out from a narrow stable of favorite foods can be challenging at first. A strategy that works well is what I call Gateway Foods.

Each child will have their own set of Gateway Foods, and for your 52 New Foods Challenge to be successful it's critical for you to figure out which ones they are. Gateway Foods, like blueberries for Catherine and James, are your ticket to some of the more challenging new foods for your family. Knowing that something familiar, and well liked, is part of the meal is like a culinary keystone for kids. It gives them a safe place from which to venture out, with the security of knowing they've got something on the table that they like.

Mixing the Gateway Food with other new foods is great, like adding a few slices of jícama and radicchio to your Blueberry-Mango Salad, but even serving the foods side by side and sampling a bit of each will move you in the right direction. Preparing a Gateway Food in a new way, like we did with mandarin oranges, is another easy way to break out of the rut and broaden your food repertoire. Try something as simple as adding a few "sprinkles"—sesame seeds, sunflower seeds, flaxseeds, nori flakes, or sliced almonds—to a Gateway Food, like green beans, to change it up. It gets your kids used to the idea of trying things in a new way, which is an important habit to foster.

The last thing you want to do is short-order cook. Serving a Gateway Food at each meal is your insurance policy. Your kids will eat what you've made even if they're not feeling adventurous, and even better, Gateway Foods might be the reason they are willing to try something new.

many exposures to a new food before a child may like it, which is why I suggest that you give your kids bonus points multiple times for trying the same food. It encourages lots of tasters.

As for competition among players at the table, I found that my kids reacted in very different ways. When Catherine smells competition, she runs from it like she would from freshly chopped onions. She plays for the fun of playing, not for the fun of winning. James, on the other hand, will turn anything into a competition. He will keep score. When we started playing for points at our table, he was laser-focused on beating the all-time record. Every time. Making it a game worked for both of them, but for different reasons.

Making it a game also helped me transform my role at the table, from a dictator to a facilitator. The root of those words highlights the key difference. The root of facilitator is *facile*, which means "to make easy," versus the root of dictator, *dictate*, which means "to speak or tell." I needed to make it *easy* for my kids to make their own good choices, as opposed to *telling them* what to do. Arguably, the reason why my kids were so much more willing to eat balanced meals was because I stepped out of the way and let them choose for themselves. Granted, they were choosing from within a healthy set of foods. My job was to ensure that there were enough colors on the table each night—to make it easy for them to round out their plates. Their job was to earn points by eating a healthy, balanced meal from the colors that were available. Mom facilitates. Kids choose.

How long, and how frequently, you choose to track points will depend on the unique personality of your family. For my kids, after a few months of playing with points they didn't need them anymore. They internalized the system. As we continued trying new foods each week, they shifted their focus to other aspects of our challenge—cooking foods, growing foods, and finding new foods at the market. They still loved the fun of our game, but they didn't need points to keep them going. Occasionally we needed a boost, like after a vacation, and points reappeared at our table to help us get back on track. Use points as a catalyst when you are stuck.

A chart outlining suggested points for foods and how to calculate your score can be found in Appendix B (page 289). I've also included a points value on the pages profiling each food in this book. Foods are ranked based on a combination of nutritional value and how challenging it is to get kids to eat them: Hence, asparagus (nutritious but sometimes tough to get kids to eat) is worth more points than apples (nutritious but relatively easy to get kids to eat).

Give Rewards

The issue of points and rewards is a thorny one. Like an arrow, it fires straight at the heart of the debate about intrinsic versus extrinsic motivation. Does your kid want to eat healthy foods because you are giving him points? What happens when the points go away? Will he cease to eat healthy when there is no tangible reward? I firmly believe that making healthy eating a game allows you to leverage extrinsic motivation to tap into intrinsic motivation.

How to Set Goals

If you run into problems, try working in reverse. Start this challenge by discussing what would be a great reward for taking on the first thirteen foods. Maybe a day trip to a favorite family destination, like the beach or your local state park. Or time with friends you don't see very often. Refer to What to Give as Rewards on page 18 to generate ideas.

Gamification, or the idea that game techniques can be applied to real-life situations, is spreading rapidly and can be skillfully applied at your family table to make healthy eating fun for everyone involved.[1] It's not just kids who benefit from the fun of a game. As parents, we benefit a tremendous amount, too. Kids (and adults) may start out a challenge because of the allure of points or a prize (leveraging extrinsic motivation), but they will only stick with it if the activity is fun in and of itself (tapping into intrinsic motivation). And the more they stick with it, the more their bodies will crave healthy foods (as opposed to foods that are engineered to make us want more[2]). They'll be more open to trying new things. It's a positive, reinforcing cycle.

My kids are a good example of how this plays out. When we first started playing Crunch a Color, it was all about the points and prizes. Inevitably the dinner discussion turned to how many points each person had racked up, who had the all-time highest points total, or which person had the most multiples for trying new foods. But as we continued to play, and eating colorful, balanced meals became second nature, my kids' focus turned away from the points and toward the sheer fun of the game. Extrinsic motivation got them over the hurdle; intrinsic motivation kept them going. The most salient example is the launch of our 52 New Foods Challenge in and of itself. My kids were craving the bigger goal and were carried forward purely for the love of the adventure. Not the points.

Critics of my game-based approach will argue that points are not much different than prizes and that a parent should not reward a child for eating, of any kind. The question is, how do you get out of the starting gate when you're at a complete standstill? I'd argue the answer is points. When points make it easier to be a good parent, and for kids to eat their colors, the points are a good thing. Points turn bad when they can be redeemed for cupcakes. Or money. Leveraging the love of a game to make healthy eating fun is a lot different than packing plastic toys in your carryout meals.

Set up rewards that encourage healthy family time together and are appropriate given your goal. Keep rewards closely tied to the action that you want your child to take—ones that reinforce a healthy lifestyle. Do not use food or money as rewards.

Tailor rewards based on the personality of your family. If your kids need immediate feedback, give a small reward for meeting your points target on your New Food Day. Small rewards for small goals. Give something simple like extra outdoor playtime on a weeknight. Stickers or sports cards can work as well. Work toward giving a reward for a month's worth of meeting your points goal on each New Food Day. Offer bigger prizes for bigger goals, like a family outing to a favorite park or beach. Download a free reward chart from my website, www.52newfoods.com, to track your progress.

Prizes aren't necessary. For many kids, the fun is in the game. A helpful comparison is to think about a game like Sorry! or chess. No prizes are awarded to the winner.

The Core Principles

Before you start your 52 New Foods Challenge, I want to share the core principles of your New Foods Plan. They are the essential ingredients that will help you catalyze deep changes and establish healthy habits that will serve your children for a lifetime. These core principles are baked into every step of the 52 New Foods Challenge. Each week presents an opportunity to practice some or all of the principles, keeping you moving along the road to mastery.

These principles may not be new to you—many of us know what we should be doing to be consistently eating in a healthy way. But why, then, aren't all of us doing it? Bringing these lessons to life at your table is what's hard, especially for a busy family. The 52 New Foods Challenge is designed to help you easily put these principles into practice.

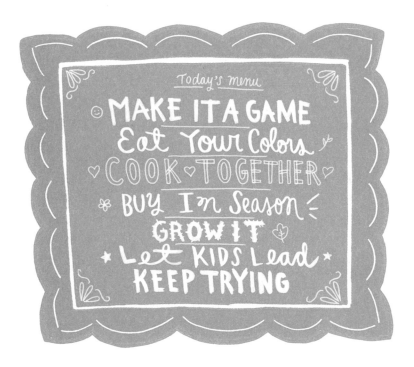

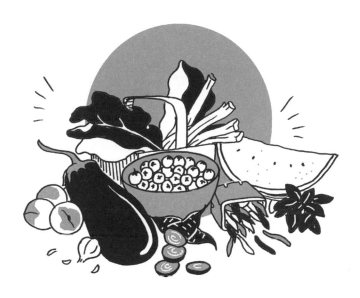

Eat Your Colors

Eat food. Not too much. Mostly plants.

—MICHAEL POLLAN

LOOKING BACK, IT WAS EASY TO SEE WHY WE NEEDED TO ADD MORE COLOR TO OUR PLATES. They were bleak and dominated by the three Ps: pasta, pizza, and peas. It didn't take a nutritionist or doctor to tell me that we needed more color in our diet. That was terribly obvious. But wouldn't it have been sufficient to get my kids to eat a few bites of broccoli every day? A few crunches of carrots? Isn't that good enough?

The answer is no. Eating broccoli is good, but eating broccoli alone does not equate to a healthy diet. And most of us don't eat enough broccoli anyhow (or any other vegetable, for that matter). According to the President's Council on Fitness, Sports, and Nutrition, most Americans do not eat the recommended amounts of fruits and vegetables. What you need is variety. Color is key, but not just one color.

You need all of the colors.

> Another way to think about this: Colors in your diet are like instruments in a symphony—the more you have, the richer the experience.

To uncover why colors are so important, and how they play a role in a healthy diet, I went straight to the experts. First, I talked with Dr. Walter Willett, the nutrition chair at Harvard University's School of Public Health and one of the nation's leading authorities on healthy eating. I asked Dr. Willett how colorful foods play a role in our health, especially the health of our children, and he reinforced the notion of diversity on our dinner plates.

> Variety is a key to nutrition. It reduces the chance of missing out on something important and also reduces the chance of getting too much of something undesirable. By aiming for a wide range of color, we help insure variety, and it also makes good nutrition appealing.

The other important distinction is in referring to food as colors as opposed to vegetables. Dr. Willett hinted at this idea when he talked about making good nutrition appealing. A colorful plate is much more exciting and enticing than a white one.[1] But there is something more when it comes to engaging kids at the table—to making healthy food appealing. The word *color* is a treasured part of a child's vocabulary. It evokes feelings of fun and playfulness and messy adventures at preschool. Kids get it, immediately, when you talk about colors. You're speaking their language. Talking about vegetables, on the other hand, can often induce fear, resistance, and a heavy dose of upturned noses.

It's marketing. Use it to your advantage.

Frances Largeman-Roth, a registered dietician, author of *Eating in Color*, and fellow mom, explains how intensity of color also plays an important role in a healthy, colorful diet:

> Brightly colored fruits and vegetables contain plant chemicals called phytochemicals (or phytonutrients). Many phytochemicals have antioxidant properties, which means they can scavenge free radicals in the body and prevent free radical damage. Our bodies are assaulted daily by free radicals, from the air we breathe, to the effects of

exercise, to pollution and the sun's rays. So we need to pack our diets with antioxidants daily. In addition to brightly colored fruits and veggies, grains, nuts, and seeds also contain antioxidants. And yes, a purple potato does contain more antioxidants than a white one. And red onions have more flavonoids than white or yellow varieties.

Hence, purple potatoes are worth more points than white potatoes.

Tips to Make It Easy to Eat Your Colors

Be a Good Facilitator

Your role as a parent is to facilitate. That means your job is to set your family up for success (make the colors available) and encourage everyone to keep trying (cheer them on). Invite your kids into the game with questions like, "How many colors can you eat tonight?" or "How would you make a meal with all of the colors on the table?" Remember, you are part of the game as well. Model good behavior by loading your plate full of colors, too, and try something new. Use Gateway Foods (page 14) so that you don't need to be a short-order cook.

Stock Up

When you shop, challenge your kids to fill the cart with colors. Aim for at least one food from each of the five color groups: green, red, yellow/orange, blue/purple, and white/brown. When you're starting out, you may find your cart is heavily weighted toward one color. In my case, it was green: green apples, green peas, and green beans. When this happens, choose your favorite foods but in a new color. For example, try purple beans instead of green ones, orange sweet potatoes instead of white russets, or red carrots instead of orange carrots. Within each color, aim for the highest intensity: Light green butter lettuce is good—deep green kale is better. Having a wide variety of colors in your fridge will be important so that you can easily feature three colors on the table each night.

Plan Your Meals

Plan for two colors at your main meal and one color for dessert. For example, try Brussels Sprouts Chips (green) and Crispy Sweet Potato Fries (yellow/orange) as sides with your main meal, and offer Warm Cinnamon Apples (red) for dessert. If you don't have much time to cook, simply chop up fresh veggies and offer them with a dip. Sliced rainbow carrots are one of my go-to colors when I'm short on time. Just get those colors on the table! This takes a bit of planning at first, but after a few weeks, you'll find it has become a healthy habit.

Dessert Can Be Colorful, Too

Serve colorful fruits for dessert on weeknights. Save sweet, healthy treats, which you make at home with your kids, for weekends if you choose to eat them. This not only boosts colors at your table but also has the added benefit of reducing added sugars in your child's diet (see page 39).

Give a Simple Formula

Use a simple formula for building a balanced meal that is easy for everyone in the family to remember: 3 colors + 1 protein + 1 healthy grain + 1 liquid = a winning plate. No soda. If you choose to track points, aim for at least 30 at each meal. The points system is outlined in Appendix B on page 289.

Keep Colorful Foods within Reach

The easier it is to reach for colorful foods, the easier it will be for your kids to choose colorful foods. Keep low shelves and drawers in your fridge stocked with prewashed, precut veggies and fruit in glass containers. This will help at snack time (and when packing lunches). A bowl of seasonal fruit on the table is another great call to action for your kids.

Be Flexible

Think about your colors over the course of the week as opposed to at just one meal. Don't stress if you don't hit your goal at each meal. It's not a straight line. The key is to keep trying. Looking at your family's eating habits over the course of a week will give you a much better view than looking at any one meal, and it will relieve the stress of worrying about whether they ate their broccoli today. You also need to be realistic in situations when it's hard to eat your colors. Being the mom who harps on healthy eating at the pizza party is a tough role to play. Remember that one "bad" meal won't erase a week's worth of good ones. In those moments, let your kids know that it's okay to make an exception and that you'll get back on track at your next meal together.

Be Smart About Food Storage

When possible, choose glass or BPA-free containers for storing your food. BPA, or bisphenol-A, is a chemical used in plastics and cans. According to the FDA, there is "some concern about the potential effects of BPA on the brain, behavior, and prostate gland in fetuses, infants, and young children."[2]

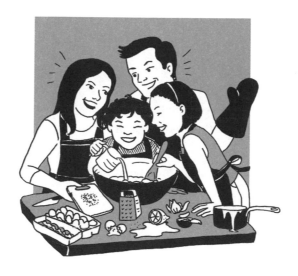

Cook Together

The only real stumbling block is fear of failure.
In cooking you've got to have a what-the-hell attitude.
—JULIA CHILD

IF YOU'RE LIKE ME (OR ANY BUSY PARENT, FOR THAT MATTER), THE THOUGHT OF COOKING together with your kids evokes one or all of the following reactions:

"It takes too much time to cook with my kids."

"Cooking with my kids is messy, which makes more work for me (and I'm already over-loaded)."

"I can get it done faster if I just cook it myself."

I know these arguments well because I used to make them.

You are right. At first, it will take more time—time that you feel you don't have to spare. It will be messier. It will be more work for you. But consider this: Time "wasted" today is quality time gained later. As your kids become more proficient in the kitchen, and together you learn to cook as a family, the health of your family will improve, your children will become more independent, and ultimately you will gain time.

Cooking together will make your life easier.

Before we started our 52 New Foods Challenge, I did most of the weeknight cooking myself, shooing the kids into the yard to play with friends (or worse, to watch TV or play on the computer) while I got dinner on the table. Cooking projects were saved for leisurely weekend days when I didn't have the pressure of a busy weeknight schedule, and when I was in a good mood. Even then, weekend cooking projects were structured in a way to segment kid-friendly steps from adult-only steps—and most of the recipes had adult-only steps! The perfectionist in me was comfortable with this clear division of labor, particularly liking that I could control most of the outcome of the dish and the corresponding mess.

An example: pancakes. In my mind, pancakes were the perfect weekend recipe to "cook" with my kids. Without the rush of a typical weekday morning, I would saunter down to the kitchen in my pajamas, brew a piping-hot pot of coffee, and enjoy the peaceful pleasure of piecing together the ingredients for our recipe—by myself. My mind would comfortably settle into autopilot, like the feeling you get when driving to a familiar destination and you arrive not realizing how you got there. A scoop of flour, measured carefully over the container to avoid scattering a faint dusting of white on the newly cleaned floor. Baking powder, baking soda, and salt, tidily placed in a little glass bowl and perched on the side of my favorite wooden cutting board. An egg, cracked and lightly beaten. Milk at the ready in a no-spill cup. Butter, melted and cooled just slightly. With my recipe prepped, everything in its place, I would beckon the kids to the kitchen to "cook." A more accurate description of the activity would be "assemble." The whole process would take less than five minutes, and leave my kids asking, "Really? Is that all? Daddy lets us do more!" With a manufactured smile, the one reserved for awkward parenting moments, I would respond, "Yep! Thanks for helping. I'll call you when it's ready." No invitation to create, no experimenting, and very little (if any) quality time together. My husband, Anthony, might let them stand at the hot stove and flip pancakes, but not on my clock!

Peering over the mixer—an arm's length away from the action—or simply assembling premeasured ingredients, didn't count as cooking together. The amount of real learning they absorbed through this observation was limited. And that learning, I realized, was the key that I needed to get my family to the next level. Beyond that, there was another very real

The Importance of Learning to Cook

As my interest in how to make healthy changes for my family grew, I began reading about how the rates of home cooking were in severe decline (and even worse, dominated by the microwave), how kids were no longer learning this basic life skill (at home or at school), and how that decline (coupled with an increase in the consumption of electronic media) was having a tremendously negative impact on the health of our kids. I was startled by the data showing the alarming increase in processed foods as a portion of the average American's weekly food purchases (nearly doubling in total dollars spent over the last thirty years),[1] and that roughly half of our budgets were being spent on food consumed outside the home (up a noticeable amount from my childhood experience, when about one-third of the average American weekly budget was spent on food consumed outside the home).[2] All of these factors were playing a role in high rates of obesity and the stark reality that this is the first generation of kids that might not outlive its parents.[3] The data was mounting. The path was gloomy, though not surprising. A big part of the solution: teach kids how to cook wholesome, nutritious foods.

reason to make a change. My kids weren't all that interested in my version of cooking anymore. Invitations to cook together were met with lukewarm interest, at best.

I had to let go of perfect and make time to learn to cook *with* my kids, not *for* my kids.

It's funny how just that one small change in preposition resulted in a big shift in my perspective. Instead of worrying about whether the portion of flour in the apple crumble was just right, or whether the pancake batter was being stirred gently enough to elicit light and fluffy flapjacks, I had to let my kids experiment. I had to learn how to invite them into the kitchen instead of pushing them away. Instead of aiming for the perfect recipe and a pristine kitchen to go along with it, I needed to encourage my kids to get their hands in the mix (literally) and fail early and often in the kitchen. It occurred to me that cooking is a great way to develop resiliency and creativity—both in my kids and myself. But how exactly was I going to do that when I could barely keep it together to get a healthy meal on the table?

My husband, Anthony, was my inspiration. Unlike me, Anthony is relaxed about everything in the kitchen, including cooking with the kids. He's by no means a chef, but he enjoys cooking and finds great relaxation in spending an hour (or more) whipping up something for everyone to enjoy. Unflappable is a good way to describe his personality, which tends to be the right mix with kids and cooking.

He started cooking together with both Catherine and James well before their respective second birthdays. If they could hold a fork and stand unassisted, Anthony had them at the stove. Toddlers and water are a match made in heaven, so washing the veggies and fruit for our family meals was always great fun. But Anthony also invited the kids to stir the eggs in the frying pan, flip the pancakes on the griddle, or season the chicken noodle soup. Harmless as these activities seem, I resisted every step of the way, convinced that someone was going to lose a digit or get scorched. I had to put my foot down on the day I walked into the kitchen to find Catherine, at the tender age of three, balanced precariously on a wobbly wooden stool, sautéing mum mums (aka mushrooms) for an omelet, while James peered over the pan from the baby carrier on Anthony's chest. Cooking with a child in the baby carrier was where I had to draw the line. To say that I was an overprotective mom is a bit of an understatement. Luckily, Anthony gently ignored most of my phobias and proceeded despite my nagging concerns (although he agreed not to cook with a kid in the carrier anymore).

In retrospect, I am so thankful for what he did. Anthony planted the seeds of cooking together in our kids' minds from an early age. He fed their curiosity and invited Catherine and James into the kitchen to explore and create. He laid the foundation for the cooking skills they would soon develop. And he created a special bond. I realized that the way I was approaching cooking was messing up all of the good work Anthony had done. But it wasn't too late.

At a very basic level, I knew that cooking was a life skill that I needed to teach my kids—like how to swim or brush your teeth. Even better was that cooking together might help us build a stronger family connection, inspire creativity in my kids, and make a positive change at our table. So I pulled up my bootstraps, took a deep breath, and kept telling myself we'd be better for the experience (even though I still cringed every time flour covered the counters and floor). This part of our 52 New Foods Challenge was more about me than my kids.

I encouraged my kids to mix, stir, pour, chop, and spill—letting them take the lead on our recipes. I focused on letting go and slowly learning to truly enjoy cooking with them. I thought of each meal more as a project than a product to be perfected. I encouraged them (and myself) to explore and experiment, to learn from mistakes and try again.

It's one thing for me to tell my five-year-old that cracking the egg too hard on the edge of the bowl will result in a big, sloppy mess on the counter, and an entirely different experience for him to learn that lesson firsthand, without Mom buzzing overhead like a helicopter. Leaving him to his own devices, he discovered that one of the easiest ways to remove bits of shell from cracked eggs was to use the half-shell he had in his hand. Dicing apples for a fruit salad quickly taught him that the way to avoid fruit rolling off the counter onto the floor, making fast food for our family dog, was to cut with the flat side of the fruit down on the cutting board. Our homemade granola bar recipe failed miserably at least five times—first, a crumbly mess that we repurposed as granola on our fruit parfaits; next, a batch that was too chewy and flopped on flavor; then another with too much peanut butter—before we found the right mix. I nearly gave up trying. But together, we kept experimenting, learning from (not lingering on) our mistakes, and laughing as we learned to enjoy cooking as a family. Instead of striving for perfection, I focused on exploring foods and experimenting with new ways to make a recipe or new combinations of flavors we could try. My goal was to foster curiosity and confidence.

Letting go of perfection and learning to love cooking and experimenting together made an unexpected impact on me. My stress levels started to sink and I found that cooking became a fun activity that we enjoyed together, as opposed to it feeling like a chore. Clearly this was good for me. But what really sold me on why it's so important to cook together as a family was the change in my kids.

At the budding young ages of seven and ten, James and Catherine have mastered some

Kids Don't Need Kids' Menus

Of all the mistakes I made in the early days of feeding my family, one of the biggest was the kids' menu—cooking a separate meal for my little ones. It was a slippery slope. First, I found myself leaving a portion of the pasta plain to accommodate fleeting fussiness. Then, no comingling of vegetables—stir-fries trended downward. Next, bland was best—I made only our go-to vegetables with little to no seasoning. Like the frog in boiling water, I didn't realize what was happening until it was too late.

As you journey forward in your 52 New Foods Challenge, commit to making meals that everyone can enjoy together. No kids' menu. Offer simplified versions of the dishes you serve—sauce on the side—but plan for everyone to eat the same meal. No substitutes. Inviting your kids to plan, shop for, and cook the food with you will go a long way to making this a smooth transition.

essential cooking skills. I beamed with pride when, as part of a school project, my daughter wrote, "My favorite thing to do is cook with my mom." This love of cooking has spread like mint in a vegetable garden. Inspired by a cooking playdate with friends, my daughter created her first recipe: Friendship Garden Soup (page 87). Together, my kids hosted a series of garden cooking classes at school to teach their friends how to make simple, family-friendly dishes. Compiling a book of recipes was top on their list of summer projects.

Even more than these discrete skills, my kids developed confidence in the kitchen, tapped into their innate creativity, grew a love of trying new things, and learned to appreciate wholesome, healthy foods. That confidence, creativity, and flexibility are evident beyond the kitchen, too. Trying a recipe for the first time is not unlike learning a new math or writing skill. It takes persistence, patience, resilience, and creative thinking. Cooking is another opportunity to practice starting from what you know, getting comfortable with making mistakes, experimenting, and learning from others.

Those are life lessons that are well worth a messy kitchen.

Great Recipes to Cook Together

Beginner: Healthy Crepes (page 117), Bitty Bites (page 221), Nut-Free Basil Pesto (page 230)

Intermediate: Mini Asparagus Frittata (page 178), Roasted Romanesco (page 135)

Advanced: Sautéed Brussels Sprouts with Lemon and Walnuts (page 78), Eggplant Parmesan (page 187)

Tips to Keep Your Sanity While Learning to Cook Together

Cooking together is the single most important key to healthy eating and an important part of your 52 New Foods Challenge. Making the change from cooking *for* your kids to cooking *with* your kids can feel like a big jump. The secret is to take it one small step at a time. Channel your inner Julia Child and muster up a what-the-hell attitude.

Remove Constraints

Start by setting aside a weekend afternoon to cook together, without time constraints. Try just one day a week for an hour. Together with your kids, pick an easy, healthy recipe to make, like our Bitty Bites (page 221). You can provide guidance for your kids on the types of recipes that would be a good fit, but it's important to let them choose from within that set. Set up your cooking project like an activity, with all of the supplies you need within arm's reach on the family table. Do not pre-anything: no premeasuring, precutting, prescooping, or premixing!

Let Go

With your recipe in hand and your supplies ready to go, let your kids measure, scoop, stir, and roll. Let go and let them do it. Then enjoy your dish together!

Ask them:

"What did you enjoy about making that dish? What would make it easier?"

"What would you add to that recipe?"

"What surprised you?"

"How would you teach that recipe to a friend?"

As you get comfortable, branch out into more challenging dishes. Try recipes that call for peeling, squeezing, chopping, and sautéing, like Mini Asparagus Frittatas (page 178). No need to invest in kids' cooking tools. Let them use the kitchen tools that you use, with close supervision at first. Encourage your kids to try dishes other than dessert. It's easy to lean on baking, but it's important for your kids to learn that they can have just as much fun creating a delicious soup or side dish. Cooking isn't only about cookies!

Experiment

As you and your kids become more comfortable working together in the kitchen, let them experiment with creating recipes and trying new combinations. Last summer, my kids were captivated by trying to master homemade lemonade. They experimented with different types of lemons, mashing mint and strawberries to add different flavors, and sweetening their concoction with honey. Never were they more proud to serve lemonade at their make-shift summer stand than when they made the whole thing themselves, squeezing and stir-ring with their own hands and following no other guidance than their intuition.

Get Both Parents Involved

In most families, there is one person who does most of the cooking. But it's important for *both* parents to find ways to cook with the kids. In addition to cooking together as a family on your New Food Day, encourage your partner to master (at least) one recipe that can be his or her special dish. Several recipes in this book are my husband's, including Brussels Sprouts Chips (page 77), Healthy Crepes (page 117), and Anthony's Famous Short Ribs (page 285).

They provide an easy starting point for the parent in your family who is just learning how to cook.

Some Simple tips for keeping Kids safe while Cooking

1. Wash hands first! Pick a song, like the ABCs, and sing it *twice* while you wash.

2. Work on a stable, flat surface that is an easy height for your kids. The kitchen table, or a kids' play table, often works well. Or pull a stool to the counter.

3. Encourage your kids to measure and prep all the ingredients first, before diving into the recipe. Tidy your work area as you go. Keep a kitchen towel close by for wiping hands and catching spills.

4. Make a fist or bridge when chopping to protect little fingers from big knives.

5. Cut with the flat side of the fruit or veggie down (sometimes this means Mom or Dad should make the first cut). Remind kids to cut away from themselves and others.

6. Rock, don't jump. When using a knife, teach your kids to use a rocking motion, not an up-and-down chopping motion.

7. When scooping, sifting, stirring, and pouring, work over a rimmed baking sheet. This helps contain the mess and makes it easier for you to let go and let your kids work independently.

8. Taste as you cook. Encourage your kids to taste the recipe as you go, and adjust seasonings to tweak the flavor to find the right mix for your family.

9. Have fun (but no games like ninja fighters!).

Disclaimer: Knife safety in the kitchen is important. Throughout this book I encourage you to let your kids do the chopping. In the end, though, it is your call as a parent whether your child is ready. Each child is unique. Follow their lead, and use your best judgment.

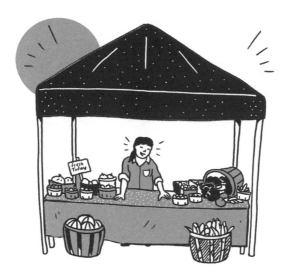

Buy in Season

Live in each season as it passes; breathe the air, drink the drink,
taste the fruit, and resign yourself to the influences of each.
—HENRY DAVID THOREAU

APPLES ARE NO LONGER AVAILABLE.

These simple words, posted on a sign at our local market, may have been small in number but they generated a big impact. Apples were the foundation of our fridge. My kids could always count on an apple if there was nothing else that they felt like eating. Even more, I could always count on an apple. What would happen if I couldn't respond to their whines and whims with "Well, then, have an apple!"?

My son, James, marched right up to the person stocking the produce and asked, "Why are there no apples?" He was befuddled. Not having apples at the market was like the sun not rising in the morning—he couldn't imagine why that would happen.

"Apples are out of season. The last batch arrived from our local grower last week, and we sold them all, so there are none left this week. Would you like to try a pear?"

This seemed like a straightforward, sensible answer. Don't we all know that apples are in season during the fall, when they take center stage with hayrides and pumpkins? Apparently not, if you primarily shop at the big-box grocery store, which is what my kids illustrated. Although some stores will prominently feature items that are in season, for the most part, the grocery store wins on consistency. It's an oasis of sameness—a happy bubble impervious to the effects of the season. As a shopper, you experience comfort knowing that you can pretty much always find an apple.

On the bright side, at least my kids were seeking out apples, not Apple Jacks. That was a win. But our apple affair made me realize that we weren't really in tune with how the seasons, or anything else for that matter, impacted what we were eating. In their worldview, food was to be consumed, color by color, and came from the store where it was in plentiful supply regardless of any outside forces (ecological or economical). My kids understood that an apple grew on a tree—that it originated in nature. Shopping the outer aisles of the grocery store didn't get them much farther than that. They didn't really understand how the road between the tree and their plates was navigated.

There was more that we had to learn.

I started by adding a layer of complexity to our weekly grocery store visits. Not only were my kids charged with finding a new food to try, but they were also challenged to find something that was in season. The telltale sign we learned to look for was the word *local*. I reasoned that if the food was grown at a nearby farm, it would be seasonally appropriate—no blackberries grown locally in California in the middle of January.

As the freeze of winter warmed into the early drops of spring, and our local farmers' market opened for business again, I started to shift our shopping to the fresh market. It took a little more flexibility on my part, mostly because I couldn't as easily plan what to shop for if we were letting the seasons be our guide. But at this point, after loosening up a bit in the kitchen, I was more willing to let go and let the adventure unfold at its own pace.

Sunday mornings, we headed down to the local farmers' market to pick our new food of the week, along with our menu for the next few days. Missing the seasonal cues at the market would be like overlooking an elephant in your living room—they were just too big to ignore. First, tender asparagus—then radiant summer squash, peas, cherries, and more. The added bonus was that we were naturally increasing our focus on whole foods, and lessening our attachment to processed foods, without any pressure from me. The only boxes at the market were the ones used to crate fresh produce. But there was another, more subtle force at work—something beyond the food.

I first noticed a shift occurring about the time that apricots arrived at the market. My kids are all about the free samples—some weeks those bites served as their breakfast—so when we arrived for our weekly visit they swarmed the fruit stand like bees and happily sampled every variety available. As they munched away, the farmer sliced up a fresh batch of plumcots—a delicious cross between an apricot and a plum—to restock her reserves and then offered a few to her enthusiastic (and hungry) customers. They were hooked. The taste of this new fruit at its seasonal peak was mouthwatering.

"How can I tell which ones are the juiciest?" James asked.

"For fruit that you plan to eat today, pick the ones that are a soft orange color. Touch them gently. They should have a little bit of give," explained the farmer, showing James how to tenderly touch the fruit to test for ripeness. James went to work, carefully selecting his treasure and placing it gently in his tattered woven bag.

"Be sure to pick a few that are green near the top," the farmer advised. "Those will be perfect in a day or two if you leave them on the counter to ripen."

While James was occupied packing his bag full of fruit, Catherine found her opportunity to join the conversation. "How do you like to cook them?" she asked.

The farmer seemed to drift off into a happy place, as though she was daydreaming about the myriad ways she liked to prepare her bounty. She replied, "My favorite is to eat them when they're fresh picked, but it is also a wonderful treat to bake them with honey and pistachios. I also love to make jam. That might be fun for you to try. Let me know what you make, and how it turns out."

Like a good teacher, the farmer had given my kids a few ideas to work with and then encouraged them to run with them and report back with their findings. The next time we visited the market, Catherine and James sought out the apricot farmer, not only to stock up on her delicious fruit but also to share news of what they had made—it was the inkling of a friendship.

A similar encounter happened when okra arrived at the market a few weeks later. A favorite food for Catherine, she raced to fill her basket as if she were collecting candy at a carnival. As she rummaged, I asked the farmer, "Where is your farm located?"

"About four hours from here," he replied, without the faintest note of strain in his voice.

He drove eight hours a day, three days a week, to bring his produce to market. "We were up before the sun this morning."

Catherine's eyebrows rose in two perfect arches and she whispered to me, "That's a really long drive." I nodded in agreement, thinking how often I complained about driving to hockey practice at 7:00 a.m., which seemed soft in comparison. It was beginning to register, for all of us, that it wasn't an industrial machine that brought healthy food to our table. It was often a person, who worked hard and took pride in the food that he or she grew.

We got an even greater sense of that hard work in the strawberry fields. Buckets in hand, we followed the rows upon rows of berry bushes out to the sun-drenched fields. Crouched low to the dusty ground, Catherine and James spent the better part of our morning picking fresh berries—strawberries, blackberries, and if they were lucky, the occasional olallieberry. With stained fingers as proof of their effort, they harvested a mere two buckets of berries. It was barely more than what we would buy on a typical visit to the market, but earned the hard way.

In the thick of our 52 New Foods Challenge, it was difficult to pinpoint how buying in season at our local farmers' market, or picking it straight from the vine, was altering our outlook on food. Aren't vegetables—conventional or not, local or not—better than a cupcake? We were eating our colors, we were cooking and exploring foods together, but looking back I realize that tuning into the seasons by getting to know our local farmers was about more than the food.

Taste was a factor. The locally grown foods we were eating were often fresher than what we found at the grocery store and, in most cases, tasted better. This was highly evident with strawberries—the watery flavor of a basket of berries from the grocery store compared to the juicy ripe flavor of our peak-picked local berries was dramatic—but most anything we ate at the peak of its season from the fresh market simply tasted better, which in turn made it easier for my kids to try it. But shopping locally, or picking it with our own hands, helped us move beyond thinking just about ourselves to thinking a little more broadly—to the land that was growing our food and the farmers who were tending and harvesting it. Shopping locally reaffirmed our decision to choose sustainably raised food to help care for the environment, even if our view of that environment was simply the land immediately surrounding us.

The importance of choosing seasonal, locally grown, sustainably farmed foods is something I could teach my kids (and myself), dutifully. But for us to *believe it*—and not just regurgitate it like well-trained school children—we had to *feel it*.

It was the community—the interactions with people—that nurtured that feeling. The conversations we had with the farmers each week—hearing what they were growing, getting tips on how to prepare the foods that they harvested, and sharing with them what we had made with their bounty—helped to build a connection beyond palate or politics. We became part of a community.

Teach Your Kids to Read Food Labels

When shopping with your kids, your focus will be on whole fruits and vegetables (or foods that don't come in a box or have a label). But the reality of the supermarket is you will encounter foods that come in a package, so you need to have a plan in place to deal with it. The solution: Teach your kids to read food labels to know what's in the food you're eating.

Rule #1: The fewer words the better, and sugar shouldn't be one of the first five.
Rule #2: If you can't read the words on the label, put it back on the shelf.

As for my rising third grader, who was apt to sound out her words, I tacked on a rider, "Or if it's something you wouldn't find in nature." I didn't think she was growing a fructo-oligosaccharide plant in the school garden.

Added Sugars

The FDA is proposing a change to food labels, making it easier to calculate the number of "added sugars," noted in grams (for reference, 4 grams = 1 teaspoon). Added sugars include refined white sugar, honey, maple syrup, agave, and brown sugar (among other natural, but added, sweeteners).[1] It does not include naturally occurring sugars like the ones found in whole fruits and vegetables. It is shocking how quickly added sugars can escalate if you're not watching closely. Currently, the World Health Organization recommends limiting added sugars to 10 percent of an adult's caloric intake, but at the time of writing this book there is talk of dropping that limit to 5 percent. That would put the average nine-year-old at a maximum of five teaspoons of added sugar a day (that's roughly twenty grams).[2] A can of soda can be two times that amount in many cases.[3] Don't be fooled by juice either—some juices can easily pack more than five teaspoons in a ten- to twelve-ounce serving.[4] The fastest way to cut out added sugars from your family's diet is by eliminating sweetened beverages, like soda and juice. Choosing fruit for dessert on weekdays, instead of sweet treats, will also help reduce added sugars in your child's diet. Use unrefined sweeteners, like honey, in moderation, and make your treats at home to give you more control.

> **A Word About GMOs**
>
> GMOs, or genetically modified organisms, are creating a great deal of debate in the national food conversation. According to the World Health Organization, GMOs "are organisms in which the genetic material (DNA) has been altered in a way that does not occur naturally." Although you can find arguments on either side of this debate, for me, it was a purely emotional decision. A food modified to tolerate pesticides is one that I'd like my family to avoid when possible—a personal choice. GMOs are an issue that I would encourage you to research thoroughly, talk about with your family, and decide on together. Above all, I urge you to knowingly make the choice, with eyes wide open. Certified organic produce is GMO-free. But for the times when the food we eat comes in a package, we rely on a little blue and green box—the Non-GMO Project Label—to distinguish whether GMOs are present or not.

Tips to Buying in Season

Your food is part of a community (whether you recognize it or not). Getting to know that community helps you get to know your food and leads you to make more informed choices. This shift—from consumption to community—was one of the key factors in changing the way that my family thinks about food.

Buy in Season at the Grocery Store

Start by making a small change to the way you shop at your regular grocery store, and aim for the majority of your purchases to be in season. The 52 New Foods list is a great place to start (page 61)—the foods are organized by season. Buy apples in the fall, grapefruit in the winter, tomatoes in the summer. Forgo fruits and vegetables that aren't in season, even if they are available. During the growing months in your community, choose locally harvested, organic produce whenever possible to enjoy the season's best and support your local food community. That said, having grown up in Canada, I understand how challenging it can be to find locally grown, seasonal produce during the winter. Try to choose seasonal even if it's not local—for example, enjoy watermelon in the summer months *only*, even though it's in your grocery store in December.

> Your goal is to minimize "airplane food" as much as possible— that is, food flown in from a different hemisphere.

Make the Farmers' Market a Regular Part of Your Shopping Routine

When spring arrives, plan to shop your local farmers' market on a regular basis. Once a month is a good start. Try to work your way up to once a week. Head out together as a family and encourage everyone to find something new that you can cook together. Resist the temptation to plan your menu ahead of time and try to choose foods based on what inspires you and your kids at the market. When we started shopping the local farmers' market, we focused on finding at least one new food to try for our weekly challenge. When you're ready for a bigger challenge, make an entire meal with ingredients sourced exclusively from your local farmers' market.

Make an effort to strike up a conversation when you're at the market. Start by asking the farmer, "What do you want to eat today?" Farmers know what is best at the market each day, and they might help you tune in to a new food that you haven't tried.

Build In Time

Shopping with the seasons and at the local farmers' market means you'll be naturally purchasing fewer processed or packaged foods. As a result, you may find that you have to shop more frequently—without preservatives your food may not last as long as you're used to.

Eat the Leaves First

If you can shop only once a week, make your food last by using this strategy: Eat the leaves first. Plan your weekly menu to start with foods that grow above the ground, like kale, lettuce, and other leafy vegetables, which will spoil first. Eat foods that grow below the ground at the end of your week, e.g., roots like carrots and sweet potatoes. Those will last longer.

Keep Your Food Budget in Check

Eating healthy can be expensive, particularly when organic foods are involved. To keep our food budget in check, I follow these five simple guidelines.

1. **Carrots Are Better than Candy.** A conventional carrot is better than a candy bar. We could argue the merits of organic foods, but in the end you'll do better choosing the carrot: conventional or not.

2. **Choose the Clean Fifteen.** When eating conventionally grown produce, choose the Clean Fifteen. According to the Environmental Working Group,[5] the following foods have fewer pesticide residues: asparagus, avocados, cabbage, cantaloupe, cauliflower, sweet corn, eggplant, grapefruits, kiwi, mangoes, onions, papayas, pineapples, sweet peas, and sweet potatoes. Save your budget to choose organic, when possible, for the Dirty Dozen (Plus): apples, celery, cherry tomatoes, cucumbers, grapes, hot peppers, nectarines (imported), peaches, potatoes, spinach, strawberries, sweet bell peppers, kale/collard greens, and snap peas (imported). These foods tend to be high in pesticide residue. There is much research to be done on the impact of pesticides, but in the end, I just feel better choosing organic for my kids and the environment.

3. **Shop Sales.** Look for organic, seasonal produce that is *on sale*. Buy extra and freeze a few servings for later. If it's not on sale, try not to buy it.

4. **Eat Less Meat.** Meat can be expensive, especially when it's organic. Start with one meat-free day a week, like Meatless Monday.

5. **Prepared Foods = Leftovers.** Prepared foods, whether from the hot counter at your grocery store or a box in your freezer, are costly. Make leftovers your "prepared foods" of choice. When you cook, prepare extra and save it for when time is tight.

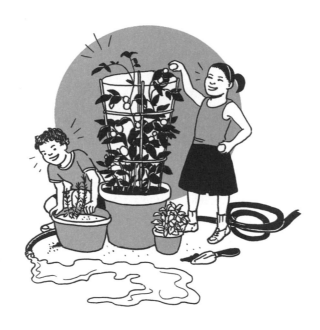

Grow It

More grows in the garden than the gardener sows.
—OLD SPANISH PROVERB

"I TRIED CAULIFLOWER TODAY," CATHERINE EXCLAIMED, AND WITH A NOTE OF SURPRISE SHE continued, "and I liked it!" She bounced into the car with an uncharacteristic late-afternoon energy—notable since most afternoons at pickup my kids flopped around like rag dolls with merely a grunt as a greeting.

A series of questions flooded my mind. Was it something she tried from a friend's lunchbox? Or was it something new that appeared on the cafeteria menu that someone convinced her to try? I had attempted to get Catherine to eat cauliflower countless times, to no avail. I must have paused too long running scenarios in my head, so Catherine piped up, "We harvested it from the garden this afternoon. I tried beets and onions, too. We baked them on our garden pizza!" A huge smile came over my face. Not only was I happy that Catherine had tried these previously blacklisted foods, but she had also experienced all of this without my help.

"That's fantastic!" I cheered. "Will you show me what you are growing?"

Instead of racing home, I parked and together we headed down the rocky trail to the school garden. With confidence, Catherine gave me and James a tour of what was growing in the raised beds—kale and lettuces, strawberries and rhubarb, onions and beets. She showed us what was ready to harvest and what was waiting in the wings. She helped James feed the resident chickens, advising him to pick strawberry leaves since they were a house favorite. Peeking into the henhouse, she spotted three fresh eggs, a reward for her class's hard work.

The connection she made with her school garden didn't stop there. For the next several weeks, Catherine continued to spend her free time at recess tending the garden and tasting the literal fruits of her labor. She taught me how to make strawberry-rhubarb crisp and shared her tips for how to grow onions. She tried fava beans and cucumbers. She discovered for herself that she preferred cauliflower raw as opposed to roasted, and made that simple request whenever cauliflower was on our menu. Taking the lead at home, she encouraged us to plant more vegetables in our growing kitchen garden.

This was the boost I needed for our ambitions to grow a meal. Months earlier, we had started a small kitchen garden and had been attempting to grow (some of) our own food. Although my kids were very excited about this project, I was deeply skeptical. Not only did I wonder how I was going to fit gardening into our already jam-packed weekly schedule, but I was notorious for being unable to grow anything. When we landscaped our yard, I picked exclusively drought-tolerant plants. After countless attempts at growing orchids, among other basic houseplants, my husband, Anthony, invested in fake blooms. My track record in this arena was weak. Very weak.

So I started small.

A gaggle of abandoned flowerpots provided us with an adequate starting place. Our local market offered a small selection of herbs and easy-to-grow vegetables, perfect for the beginning gardener, so I let my kids pick the ones that piqued their interest. Together we decided that a few kitchen staples like basil, parsley, rosemary, and mint would do the trick. Tomato plants were in abundant supply at the time, so we decided to add those to our list as well. I had seen all of these plants growing at our preschool years before, so I reasoned that if a three-year-old could grow them, certainly I could figure it out. We spent the afternoon filling pots with fresh soil, snuggling our seedlings into their beds, watering gently, and assembling our new "garden" on the stairs leading from our deck to the backyard—a sunny spot that we passed each day. I hoped that frequent, casual encounters would provide a necessary reminder to water and tend to our new plants. As for the tomatoes, we gave them a home in an unoccupied raised bed, one that had been more of a sandbox than a vegetable garden, thinking they needed some room to stretch their vines.

As the weeks passed, our little kitchen garden seemed to grow into a part of our daily routine. Unlike my unsuccessful attempts at trying to get Catherine to walk, feed, and brush our dog, Charley, I would often find her happily tending the garden—pruning dried leaves, watching for new growth, and watering diligently—without any prompting from me. James became our chief tomato inspector, initiating daily rounds to investigate developments and spot the first signs of fruit.

Our plants were growing on us.

Occasionally, we would add a few sprigs of fresh herbs to one of our dishes. My requests to head out to the backyard to find something to add to a recipe were generally met with enthusiasm. Rosemary started making regular appearances in our favorite roast chicken dish, the kids began experimenting to find the optimal mix of mint and fresh lemons for their lemonade, and we used the basil to make a delicious pesto. James fell in love with that pesto recipe, not only for the taste but because it was great fun harvesting the raw materials and blending them up in the food processor. He beamed with pride each time his pesto was featured on our table and was even more proud when he taught his friends at school how to make it. I wouldn't say that we had transformed into gardeners, but we were moving in the right direction.

Our small kitchen garden was a good start, the proverbial toe in the water, but the school garden coupled with our efforts at home really brought it together, for all of us.

"It's the difference between being told to do something and deciding to do it yourself," Curt Ellis, cofounder of FoodCorps, told me when we talked about what happens when kids grow their own food. "If a grown-up says, 'Eat your vegetables!' it isn't engaging. But if it's the child's idea, if they grow that vegetable, then suddenly, the kids are the ones with pride."

There are certainly plenty of studies to show that kids who grow their own food are more likely to try new foods and eat healthier foods in general.[1] But a garden offers more than just getting kids to move beyond peas and pasta. A garden, regardless of its size, offers kids a special opportunity to connect with nature—to learn, in a hands-on way, about where their food comes from and how it impacts our health.

Which brings me back full circle to Catherine's willingness to try cauliflower. Whether it's the promise of your kids trying something new, or building a sense of independence, or the potential health benefits from exposure to dirt and microbes, a garden plays an important role in your 52 New Foods Challenge. Let nature work its magic.

Tips to Grow a Simple Kitchen Garden

You don't need to grow a restaurant-quality kitchen garden, or have access to a school garden, to enjoy growing a meal with your kids. The key is to start small. If I can do this, as a person who is notoriously bad at maintaining anything, you can do this!

Dedicate Space

Dedicate a small patch of soil for a kitchen garden. Even an indoor planter box or colorful pots will do.

Start with Staples

Begin by focusing on easy-to-grow kitchen staples like lettuce and herbs. I am a terrible gardener, but there are a few simple crops, like basil and butter lettuce, that I can count on even when I neglect them. I've found it easiest to use starter plants, though it is fun to experiment with growing seeds, even if they don't make it. Start seeds in an empty cardboard egg carton. When (or in my case, if) the seedlings grow, transfer the plants to larger pots or a raised bed.

Plant Your Colors

As you build confidence, round out your garden with vegetables like zucchini, tomatoes, and cucumbers. The same principles that we use for colorful meals at dinner can be applied in the garden. Plant your colors—red tomatoes, green basil, yellow summer zucchini, purple radicchio, and white onions.

Start in the Spring

Expert gardeners will argue that you can grow something in each season, but as a beginner I found the summer months to be the easiest. Summer growing means that in the early spring, you should plan out which vegetables and herbs you'd like to try growing. Know that some of what you plant won't make it. Be flexible and chalk it up to learning for the next time. In midsummer, plant another few pots of fresh basil, for example, to keep things rolling into early fall. If you're inspired to try your hand at growing something in the winter months, fill a window box with small pots of herbs and keep it in a sunny location in your kitchen so you can easily add a touch of "garden fresh" to your winter soups.

Think Seed to Table

Feature one vegetable or herb from your garden on your dinner menu each week through the summer months. Put the kids in charge of harvesting and preparing the dish. I employ a highly liberal definition of a garden-grown meal—one that favors busy parents and bad gardeners! Even the simple act of harvesting and adding fresh herbs to one of your dishes will begin to build this important connection.

Call a Friend

You know that special person who has a knack for growing anything? My good friend Kathie is that person. For Kathie, unlike me, gardening comes easily. As we were testing recipes for this book, Kathie was my go-to source for garden-fresh veggies and fruit. She regularly supplied baskets of fresh herbs, handfuls of fresh lavender, lemons by the dozen, and bushels of zucchini. In return, we delivered homemade lavender cookies, fresh lemonade, and zucchini muffins. What you need is a Kathie. Call a friend and ask if you can help them harvest their bounty. They will welcome the extra sets of hands. Then cook up a delicious dish and make enough to share. For a gardener, seeing their work come full circle is a wonderful gift.

Start a School Garden

If you can rally support, start a school garden. I wouldn't dare mislead you: A school garden is not for the faint of heart. A successful school garden requires an unrelenting champion. But if you can muster a team of like-minded parents to band together, a school garden will provide much more than the vegetables that grow there. My favorite sources for school garden tips are Alice Waters' Edible Schoolyard (edibleschoolyard.org) and FoodCorps (food corps.org).

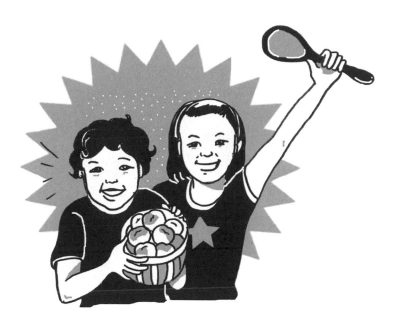

Let Kids Lead

*All children are artists. The problem is how to
remain an artist once he grows up.*
—PABLO PICASSO

THE SECRET TO MAKING THE 52 NEW FOODS CHALLENGE FUN IS TO PUT YOUR KIDS IN charge. This shift will reduce stress at the table and keep your kids engaged. But giving kids the reins offers another, even bigger benefit. Letting kids lead in the kitchen unlocks their creativity and builds confidence.

But what does it look like to let kids lead? How do you give your kids opportunities to explore while offering appropriate guidance? An experiment prompted by a basket of figs offers a great illustration of what happens when you let kids lead.

Balanced on a block of cheese was a ruddy wooden plank and two stainless-steel bowls—one containing a package of unsalted butter and the other filled with a big batch of freshly picked figs. It was an unlikely scenario in our kitchen—one that I hadn't expected when we decided to try cooking with figs.

A humble basket of figs from my friend Kathie's garden initiated our food experiment. When figs arrived on our doorstep, together as a family we talked about the ways we might like to try them—a sweet fig bar recipe topped the list. The recipe called for a pound of fresh figs. Without a kitchen scale, how were we to know how many figs to use?

James was studying balance in his first-grade science class—perfect timing for our fig conundrum. He started by suggesting that we could simply hold a package of butter in one hand and a bowl of figs in the other and guesstimate. He quickly discovered it was difficult to decipher the difference between the two sides.

"We could make a scale!" he suggested, surprising even himself. "We need something long and straight for the arms." He scurried to the garage with my husband to source materials for his contraption. The oversize ruler he used in his first try proved to be too flexible, which led him to the sturdy wooden plank. A block of cheese from our fridge served as the fulcrum. With the one-pound package of butter on one end, he started adding figs to the other until he achieved the balance he was seeking: fourteen figs.

Google could have easily answered our question. Or I could have just bought a basic kitchen scale. But those solutions would have lessened the learning that was at hand. By letting James experiment, and figure out a solution for himself, he had the opportunity to learn much more than how many figs are in a pound.

George Kembel, a fellow parent and the co-founder of Stanford University's Design School (known as the Stanford d.school), was intrigued by our fig experiment. He is one of the country's leading experts when it comes to creativity. I talked with George about the essential ingredients that foster creative thinking, and how those same themes run through every activity related to food when we let kids lead. At its core, the creative process is a process of discovery. The way to unlock creative potential is to remove barriers and allow people the freedom to experiment. Although there are several parts to the creative design process taught at Stanford, George was able to distill it down to the essence: "There are two primary modes of creativity: Trying to understand the problem and then experimenting your way toward solving it. You need to give time to explore and understand before jumping in."

When it comes to food, that means giving kids time to play and explore, like figuring out how to weigh a pound of figs without a scale. The role of the parent is to set the stage for success, then step out of the way. When a recipe fails, or doesn't turn out the way we had hoped, our job is to embrace that failure, highlight the learning in the situation, and try again. For cooking to inspire creativity, you need to provide ways for kids to explore the materials—to understand a food's inherent nature, from how it is grown to how it feels, smells, and tastes—and then experiment together with ways to use those materials. Each time you experiment you learn something new, which informs your approach the next time.

Most cooking projects or programs that teach kids to cook are designed around learning a specific technique. A teacher or parent shows the child exactly how to use the knife, exactly how to follow the ingredients list, and exactly how the dish should turn out in the end. Success is the perfect pie/cake/cookie that looks like the picture in the cookbook. But if your goal is to inspire creativity, then you need to build in time for discovery and experimentation. You welcome failures as a way of learning. It's not about the perfect recipe—it's about exploring food together. There is as much value in thinking about how to get the seeds out of a pumpkin, or how to measure a pound of figs, as there is in making (and eating) those foods. This naturally happens when you let kids lead. Giving kids the opportunity to lead allows them to exercise their innate creativity and build the confidence to continue experimenting with new ways to try things. It shows them that their thinking is as important as your thinking, that failures are an essential part of the process, and that everyone learns together.

It's the recipe for growing healthy, curious kids.

Tips to Let Kids Lead

Make it your goal to use food and cooking to inspire creativity in your kids. Focusing on the process of discovery, instead of the end goal, will make it easier for you to let your kids lead. The recipes in this book reflect this fresh, new approach and are designed to inspire creativity and confidence—in the kitchen and beyond.

Let Kids Choose, and Keep It Fun

Within your season, the foods can be taken in any order. Review the 52 New Foods section of this book together (page 61) and invite your kids to choose which foods they'd like to try first. Sort the thirteen foods into two lists—favorite foods and foods to explore (ones they think they won't like). Ask, "What do you like about the foods on our favorites list?" Follow with, "What do you wonder about the foods on our explore list?" and "What gives you that idea?" Talk about textures, smells, and looks, as well as the way that your family normally prepares each food. Discuss other ways you might try those foods—roasted versus raw, boiled versus broiled. Highlight foods that *you* plan to try because *you* haven't liked them in the past. It's important for your kids to see that everyone in the family is trying something new. Keep it positive by focusing on the things you're excited about exploring, as opposed to harping on all the things that are wrong at your table. For example, say, "I'm excited to try sweet potatoes because I'd like to find ways to make our table more colorful," instead of, "You don't eat enough vegetables and I'm worried about your health!"

Don't Give All the Answers—Keep Asking

Most kids will have a lot of questions as you explore together. Instead of jumping to explain, whether it's how a particular food tastes or how it's typically prepared, try to follow your child's questions with another question. If your child asks, "What does an artichoke taste like?" follow their question with another question like, "What do you think an artichoke might taste like? What gives you that idea?" If they ask, "How do you get the seeds out of a pumpkin?" follow with, "What do you think would work best? Let's try it together!" Use their inquiries as a springboard for conversation, and to allow them space to explore and express their ideas.

Invite Exploration

Build in time for your kids to explore foods before you start cooking with them. Think about this in broad terms. Exploring foods can extend all the way back to your garden, experimenting with growing your own food (see Grow It on page 43). Other ways to explore foods include talking with farmers at your local market (see Buy in Season on page 35), asking friends and family members about their favorite recipes, or just playing with the raw materials (see Explore Foods with Your Five Senses on page 53). Provide easy access for your kids—keep fresh fruits and vegetables in low drawers in your fridge, or in a bowl on the kitchen table, in the same way that you might keep markers and crayons out on a craft table. When you cook together, work on a surface that is at the right height for your kids, which is more often the kitchen table (or a low kids' table) than the kitchen counter.

Turn Failures into Opportunities

It can be immensely frustrating when a recipe doesn't turn out the way that you intended, or you've spent a great deal of time making something together and your child won't give it a try. Reframe failures to improve what you do the next time or uncover new ways to try something. Model this by focusing on what you learned when a recipe fails instead of throwing up your hands in frustration. It's also helpful to start with easy, fast turnaround recipes so that you can try new things more quickly.

Explore Food with Your Five Senses

An easy way to let kids lead an exploration of new foods is to encourage them to use their senses. The foods below offer a bold experience in all five sensory domains: sight, smell, touch, sound, and taste. Try setting up a sensing bar, just like a tasting bar. Offer foods in their raw and cooked forms. I've suggested some questions to get you started. Remember, there are no right answers. Listen to your kids, then respond to their comments with another question, such as, "How would we test that?" or "Is that always true?" or "How is that different from the last time you tried this food?"

Garlic
Onion
Pomegranate
Grapefruit
Kale

Sight

What does the shape of this food look like to you? Where else have you seen this shape in nature? Why do you think it grows in that shape?

Smell

Which adjectives would you use to describe the smell of this food? How does the smell change when it's raw versus cooked? What do you think causes that change?

Touch

What does the skin of this food feel like? How does that compare to the feeling of the inside, when you cut it open?

Sound

Does this food make sounds? Does the skin crinkle? Hold the food to your ear and tap the outside. Where have you heard that sound before? What sound does this food make when it's cooking? Does it make a sound when you eat it?

Taste

How would you describe the taste of this food when it's raw? How does the taste change when it's cooked? How does the taste compare to the smell?

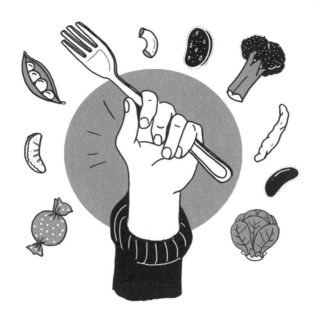

Keep Trying, Together

If you care about what you do and work hard at it,
there isn't anything you can't do if you want to.

—JIM HENSON

"I DON'T LIKE IT [TODAY]!" DOESN'T MEAN "I WON'T LIKE IT EVER!" REMEMBER THAT IT CAN take ten to fifteen exposures to a food before your child may like it.[1] And even then, they may never like it. A resistance to trying new foods is a natural phase for all children, called food neophobia.[2] It begins when kids start to walk and can continue until their teenage years—a biological safety switch designed to prevent young children from toddling off to eat a poisonous leaf. Kids also have more taste buds than adults, and those buds are tuned into sweet more than bitter, which can also contribute to challenges when tasting and trying new vegetables.[3]

The remedy? Keep trying, together.

At our family table, even putting the food in your mouth and spitting it out counts as a "taster" and earns you those coveted bonus points. When my kids resist trying something because they haven't liked it in the past, I respond with something like, "Your taste buds grow and change just like your body grows and changes. Maybe you should give it another try. You might surprise yourself!" If they don't like it (again), I offer this encouragement: "That's okay. Let's make it together another way next time. There are many different ways to prepare this food." Provide encouragement, then move on and plan to try again another day.

Build Trust

Over the course of our journey, I've talked with several nutritionists, feeding therapists, and doctors, including Dr. Alan Greene, a nationally recognized pediatrician and founder of drgreene.com. He shared this advice:

> Kids are designed to not trust new fruits and vegetables, but in certain settings that trust can change. One of the ways to do that is eating foods together as a family—you trust it more if others around you are eating it. Another way is to involve your kids. The more involved the child is in preparation of the food, the more likely it is for that trust switch to turn on.

Tips to Keep Trying, Together

This book is filled with tips on how to get your kids to keep trying new foods, but there are a few key strategies that you should know about up front.

The Work-Your-Way-Up Strategy

As with all changes, it's important to give your kids time to adjust. For example, instead of switching to whole wheat flour from refined white flour in one step, slowly shift the balance. First, replace one-quarter of the refined flour in your recipes, then half, and so on, until you're using all whole-grain flour. Shift the balance every week. It may take more than a month, and that's fine. Just keep slowly moving toward your goal. A great recipe to try this strategy with is Healthy Crepes (page 117). The Work-Your-Way-Up Strategy can also be applied to rice—work brown rice into your white rice in small, manageable increments—or pasta.

This strategy works with vegetables, too. For example, it took my kids time to warm up to the flavor of bok choy. I started by slowly working it into their favorite stir-fries and soups—a great starting point. Once Catherine and James warmed up to bok choy when it was embedded in a savory stir-fry, then we moved on to trying it solo. Having encountered this light leafy green a few times before, planted gingerly among other favorite foods, it wasn't nearly as scary when they met face-to-face.

Reliable New Food Vehicles

The stir-fry I used to introduce bok choy was one of my new food vehicles—a recipe I knew my kids would eat that could easily be tweaked to feature a new food. I used the same strategy to introduce asparagus. Starting from a basic frittata recipe that I knew my kids would eat, I experimented with letting them personalize the frittata with a few new foods—asparagus, kale, mushrooms, and broccoli.

No Sneaking!

A critical part of your food adventure involves having your kids prepare their own food to know what is in their food. No secret ingredients, hidden in the mac 'n' cheese or blended into a smoothie. If your kids are going to eat it, then make sure they peel it, squeeze it, chop it, or dice it! See Zucchini Muffins on page 183 for an example of how to put this idea into practice.

Experiment with Tastes and Textures

Catherine's experience with cauliflower is one example of why it's important to experiment with tastes and textures. We tried cauliflower roasted, sautéed, and raw. Her strong preference was for the latter. I never would have known had we not tried it lots of different ways—my preference is for roasted cauliflower and I assumed she would like it that way, too. This kind of experimentation also revealed a love of radicchio. It was Catherine's preference for crispiness that led us to slice radicchio into thin strips and roast it until it was crispy. She and James ate the entire batch straight from the pan. It was a food I never would have known that they would like had we not tried lots of different textures—now Ridiculous Radicchio Chips (page 128) are a regular on our winter menu. Same goes for Brussels Sprouts Chips (page 77). Remember that you may like a food one way, but your kids might have a preference for a different texture or flavor. Don't assume that your preference is their preference.

Take a Dip

Researchers have found that kids who don't like the bitter taste of vegetables will eat more when dips are involved.[4] That's good news for parents of picky eaters. But can we agree that ketchup and ranch dressing have had their time? I realize that these dips work, to great effect. I've accepted that ketchup isn't going away. But try a few new delicious dip options like Greek Yogurt Dip (page 82), Nut-Free Basil Pesto (page 230), and Healthy Homemade Hummus (page 278). Be sure your kids have a hand in making them, too.

DIY Dinner

A DIY dinner is a gentle invitation to try on your own terms—another great way to get your kids to try something new without the nagging. Our DIY Rainbow Salad (page 127) is a good example of how this works. Together, prepare the ingredients for your dish and arrange them on the counter in small bowls. Offer two options for each color in your recipe: in this case, carrots and strawberries for red, pineapple and mango for orange/yellow, tomatillo and avocado for green, onions and jícama for white, and radicchio and blueberries for blue/purple. Be sure to offer a few Gateway Foods (see page 14) to give your kids a safe place from which to start. Invite your kids to make one dish for themselves and two to share. Then trade. You'll be surprised what that kind of creative freedom can do for getting your kids to try something new. Mini Asparagus Frittatas (page 178) and Black Bean Burritos (page 172) work well as DIY dinners, too.

The Veggie Course

If your kids are hungry, and you serve your colors first, you'll notice a big boost in veggie intake at your family table. Serve carbs first and the reverse holds true. I call this strategy the Veggie Course. It works particularly well on busy weeknights. When preparing dinner, start the veggies first. Get your colorful sides on the table, and while your kids are munching away finish off your main dish and healthy grains. See Artichokes (page 72) for an example of how to use this strategy at your table.

Serve It Small

Encourage tasters by serving your new food in small portions. Try soup in an eggcup or demitasse. Use mini ramekins, or a mini muffin tin, to set up a new food tasting platter. Big portions will scare off reluctant children.

Walk the Talk

Set a good example by trying something new along with your kids. In interviewing experts for this book, I found it fascinating that most people had a healthy food that they didn't like at some point. But they kept trying and with time they learned to like it. Your kids are looking to you as an example. If I wasn't willing to try okra because the texture made me squirm, why would I expect my kids to give it a try?

Remember, there is learning even if they don't like it! As much as it can be frustrating to spend time cooking a dish together to find that your kids don't like what they've made, it's important to remember that they are learning something from the experience of experimenting together.

> ### Questions to Ask When Your Kids Don't Like It
> "What other ways could we try this new food?"
> "What ingredients could we add to make this recipe in a new way?"
> "What did you enjoy about making this recipe together?"
> "If you were making this food for a friend, how would you prepare it?"

For example, despite my efforts, Catherine doesn't like onions. There are times when she'll tolerate them, but, in most cases she picks onions out of her food like a bird pecking seeds. But when it comes to preparing a dish that involves onions, she is always eager to do the chopping. The reason? Onions provide a wonderful opportunity for her to work on her knife skills. She's determined to be the best "dicer" on our team, and her fruit salad is a testament to her burgeoning talent. Catherine takes more care and time making a fruit salad than I would ever consider, dicing the fruit into perfect miniature cubes, and relishing every minute.

That's valuable learning, but not the learning I had planned.

One Bag of Cheetos Will Not Hurt Them

One unhealthy meal is not going to erase all of the healthy meals your child has eaten, or will continue to eat as you venture forward together. Embrace the fact that sometimes an unhealthy treat can be delicious. Eat it and enjoy it! Just don't make it your *everyday* choice. Birthday parties, long plane rides, and holiday celebrations are all important parts of your family experience—and unhealthy treats will show up at all of these events. It's not realistic to expect anyone (including yourself) to make healthy choices every time. Banning unhealthy treats makes them all the more alluring. It's when those unhealthy treats become the default that they cause problems.

The 52 New Foods Challenge is not about being perfect. It's about constantly working to make improvements, experimenting, and enjoying the journey together. Regardless of where we stand on the food spectrum, we all have work to do and each small step moves us in the right direction. In the end, success is if you learn something new, feel more creative and open to experimentation, and have fun exploring together along the way. That's healthy.

PART 2

52 New Foods

If you run out of ideas follow the road; you'll get there.
—EDGAR ALLAN POE

Fall

Sweet Potatoes

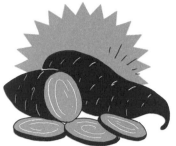

I have a weakness for fries. When we meet, I have a terrible time ignoring their unhealthy whispers. I know better. I want to set a good example. I don't want to like them, but I do. So it's not surprising to me that, as a family, we have a hard time resisting fried white potatoes with salt and a side of guilt.

But whether baked or fried, straight-up white potatoes are pretty thin when it comes to nutrition. This is a good example of a situation where color enhances the picture. Compared to their white counterparts, brightly colored orange sweet potatoes offer a substantial boost in Vitamin A,[1] and are about one-third lower on the glycemic index,[2] which indicates a lesser impact on the body's insulin and blood sugar levels (a good thing, to be sure). Baked white potatoes aren't bad, but colorful potatoes are better. Orange is more nutritious than white, and purple, if you can find them, are even more nutritious than orange.[3]

So as you add more color to your plates, look for colorful substitutes. Choose orange sweet potatoes instead of regular white russets. Our favorite way to enjoy them is to bake them like fries—the sweet flavor and crispy (just shy of burnt) texture is irresistible. Apply this same strategy to beans (try purple ones instead of green), peppers (try orange instead of yellow), or carrots (try red instead of orange). It's an easy way to make your meals more colorful and nutritious without changing much.

Make It a Game: 15 points
Eat Your Colors: Yellow/Orange

Invite Exploration

"What do you think gives orange and purple potatoes their color? What gives you that idea?"

Crispy Sweet Potato Fries

These crispy oven-baked sweet potato fries give plates a healthy boost of color. I never have to encourage my kids to try a bite of these fries. More often, I sit at the table thinking, *I should have made a bigger batch!*

PREP TIME: 10 minutes

COOK TIME: 30 to 35 minutes

Serves 4

INGREDIENTS:

2 pounds orange-fleshed sweet potatoes
(3 to 4 potatoes)

2 tablespoons extra-virgin olive oil

½ teaspoon kosher salt

Cook Together

Beginners: Peel. Toss. Arrange on the wire rack.

Experts: Cut into sticks. Parents should cut through the middle of the potato, then cut into quarters. Set the flat side down and let more experienced kids cut the sections into sticks.

DIRECTIONS:

1 Preheat the oven to 450°F.

2 Line a rimmed baking sheet with foil, then place a wire cooling rack in the pan. This makes cleanup easy and saves you from having to flip the fries partway through.

3 Wash, peel, and cut the potatoes into ½-inch-thick sticks.

4 In a large bowl, use your hands to toss the potatoes with the oil and salt.

5 Place the cut fries on the wire rack in a single, even layer.

6 Bake for 30 to 35 minutes, or until the edges are dark and crispy.

Tip *The secret to crispy fries? Cut the potatoes a little thinner than a standard French fry and bake them on a wire rack placed inside a rimmed baking sheet until the color turns to golden brown with dark edges and the skin is a little bit puffy. Serve them piping hot to avoid sogginess.*

Savory versus Sweet Fries

1 Make a batch of Crispy Sweet Potato Fries. Divide it between two medium bowls.

2 Sprinkle ½ teaspoon garlic powder and ½ teaspoon paprika into one bowl, and 1 teaspoon ground cinnamon into the other. Toss gently.

3 Serve side by side and compare.

Mashed Sweet Potatoes

Mashed sweet potatoes offer a colorful (and healthy) alternative to regular ol' mashed potatoes—plus, a way to try a new texture. They are delicious served with Easy Roasted Chicken (page 282) or Gigi's Roasted Pork Tenderloin (page 286) and a side of Brussels Sprouts Chips (page 77).

PREP TIME: 5 minutes

COOK TIME: 60 minutes

Serves 4

INGREDIENTS:

2 pounds orange-fleshed sweet potatoes (3 to 4 potatoes)

2 tablespoons unsalted butter

½ teaspoon kosher salt

DIRECTIONS:

1 Preheat the oven to 400°F. Line a rimmed baking sheet with foil or parchment paper.

2 Using a fork, prick the skin of the potatoes, making small holes all over.

3 Place the potatoes on the lined baking sheet and bake for 60 minutes, or until they are tender when pierced with a fork.

4 Let cool slightly, then halve the potatoes lengthwise (top to tip). Using a spoon, scoop out the flesh into a large bowl. Discard the skin.

5 Add the butter and salt to the potatoes. Using a potato masher, mash the potatoes until creamy. This is a fun job for cooks of all ages, but particularly well suited for kids under the age of three.

Keep Trying If your child doesn't like sweet potatoes baked like fries, try them mashed or baked whole and eaten right out of the skin. Ask, "What other ways could we try sweet potato?" or "Which other seasonings could we try with sweet potato?"

Garlic

When I asked fellow parents for tips on how to get my kids to try garlic, I felt woefully inadequate. These were the typical responses, which had me feeling hopeless:

"What's to try? Most everything we make has onions and garlic in it."

"My kids were raised with garlic being a part of everything. They don't know they don't like it."

Gold stars for everyone who started early. My kids didn't grow up with garlic and onions being an integral part of our meals. Our plates were lifeless—beaten into blandness after countless mealtime battles.

So did I give up trying to incorporate garlic into our family meals? Absolutely not! Instead of focusing on whether my kids would eat garlic, I focused on exploring and experimenting with this flavorful ingredient in lots of different ways. The secret for my kids was roasting.

Roasting garlic completely changes the smell, flavor, and texture of this simple ingredient. This is true of most vegetables, but is particularly striking with garlic. Those little white bulbs go from a piercing, burning feeling to one of warmth and softness. If raw garlic shuts you out, roasted garlic invites you in—to linger. This transformation was captivating for my kids, almost magical. It continues to delight us. If you keep exploring and experimenting with new foods, you may discover an unexpected surprise along the way.

Make It a Game: 15 points
Eat Your Colors: White/Brown or Purple

> ### Invite Exploration
>
> "Why do you think the flavor of garlic transforms when it's heated? What gives you that idea?"
>
> "What adjectives would you use to describe garlic?"

Roasted Garlic

For many kids, the taste of garlic can be overwhelming. Roasting those little white buds with a touch of olive oil transforms them into an incredibly soothing and almost sweet spread, perfect for lavishing on a crusty whole-grain loaf.

PREP TIME: 5 minutes

COOK TIME: 30 to 35 minutes

Makes 6 heads

INGREDIENTS:

6 heads garlic

1 tablespoon extra-virgin olive oil

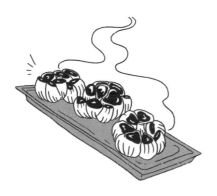

DIRECTIONS:

1   Preheat the oven to 400°F.

2   Peel away most of the flaky outer layers of the garlic bulb, but leave the head intact.

3   Cut off ¼ to ½ inch from the tops of the bulbs, exposing the inner cloves.

4   Place each head of garlic in the cup of a standard muffin tin. Drizzle each bulb with oil, then massage the oil into the cloves with your fingers.

5   Cover the pan with aluminum foil and bake for 30 to 35 minutes or until the cloves are a light brown color and soft when pressed.

6   Allow the garlic to cool, then squeeze the flesh out of the papery skin of each clove. Spread the roasted garlic on a crusty, whole-grain roll to make garlic bread.

Tip Sautéing garlic is another way to transform its flavor. The trick is to cook it quickly, just 30 to 60 seconds. If you burn it, bitterness takes over.

Cook Together

Beginners: Peel the flaky layers. Work over a rimmed baking sheet to contain the mess. Massage the oil into the bulbs. Squeeze out the cloves after roasting.

Experts: Cut off the tops.

Garlic Mushroom Toasts

This variation on garlic bread is one of Catherine's favorite recipes. Roast the garlic in advance to save time. You can serve it with or without the mushrooms, depending on your preference.

PREP TIME: 10 minutes

COOK TIME: 10 to 12 minutes

Serves 4

INGREDIENTS:

1 head Roasted Garlic
(page 69)

4 tablespoons (½ stick)
unsalted butter, at room
temperature

1 cup coarsely chopped
cremini mushrooms

Kosher salt

1 (6-inch) loaf whole wheat
French bread

Grated Parmesan cheese,
for sprinkling

DIRECTIONS:

1 Preheat the oven to 350°F.

2 Squeeze the flesh from the roasted garlic into a small bowl. Add 3 tablespoons of the butter and stir to combine. Use a potato masher if you prefer a smoother texture. Set aside.

3 In a small frying pan, melt the remaining 1 tablespoon of the butter over medium heat. Add the mushrooms and a dash of salt. Sauté for 3 to 5 minutes, or until the mushrooms are browned.

4 Slice the loaf of bread into ½-inch slices and place them on a rimmed baking sheet. Generously spread the garlic butter on each slice and top with a spoonful of mushrooms and a dash of Parmesan. Bake for 5 to 7 minutes, or until the edges of the bread are golden brown. Serve immediately.

Grow It Garlic is easy to grow in containers. Break apart the head, leave the skin on, and plant the cloves in rich, well-drained soil. Place in a sunny location. Plant in the fall, but be sure to cover when temperatures dip below freezing. Bulbs will be ready to harvest in early summer.[4]

Keep Trying Focus on exploring and cooking garlic—bonus if your kids taste it. Define success as exploring and experimenting more than eating.

Food as Inspiration

My daughter, Catherine, loves to cook. It is one of the easiest ways for me to get her to try something new at our family table. But cooking is much more than a way to increase her openness to trying new foods.

Catherine is an artist at heart, so cooking provides a wonderful opportunity for her to express herself. Creating one of her signature fruit salads is as much an exercise for her chopping skills as it is a chance to experiment with finding the right combination of colors to excite her palette. She experiences food in many different ways and with all of her senses—tasting, smelling, touching, listening, and looking.

So in addition to shopping for food together, cooking together, and growing food in our backyard, I'm always game to have her explore foods in different ways. While I was writing this book, Catherine decided to take on a writing project of her own. Recipe testing offered the perfect raw material for a series of poems and short stories—another fun way to experience some of the new foods on our list.

When a particular food we were preparing caught her imagination, she'd load up a tray of ingredients (both raw and cooked), grab her journal, and steal away to spend a few quiet minutes writing about the food we were cooking together. Occasionally a playful drawing or doodle would make it into her journal. Or a hilarious caption. But each mini writing session provided another way for Catherine to get to know the food she was eating. Writing allowed her to explore the foods we were cooking from another perspective.

Garlic

The sun reflects on the smooth marble surface
Mixing warm colors of the sky
A round globe with a pointed tip
The top of the Taj Mahal
Take it off
Turn it upside down
And spin it like a dreidel
Pick a section and peel the skin like a banana
The sharp smell catches your attention
Fire burns your tongue
Heat travels deep inside
Transforming the white skin into a pink teardrop
Inhale the warm comforting smell
A gift you can't wait to open wrapped in tissue paper
A perfect clove of garlic
Waiting to be eaten

—CATHERINE TYLER LEE, AGE 9

Artichokes

During back-to-school season, I find myself precariously balanced on the edge of having it all together and having it all fall apart. The dinner hour induces the greatest degree of this stressful feeling. Unlike my husband, who can assemble a perfectly timed meal without breaking a sweat, I find it's a struggle. Luckily for me, there is a silver lining that comes with being inept at timing. I stumbled on this strategy with artichokes.

In preparing our meal, I had forgotten to turn on the rice cooker and at serving time found an unappealing pot of cold water and wet rice. The only thing ready were the artichokes. Hunger pains were hitting their stride, so to stave off a revolt I put the artichoke on the table with a small bowl of melted butter and simple instructions: Peel, dip, eat. To my surprise, they ate all of it. The next night I tried again: veggies first, carbs and proteins second. Although not statistically significant, net veggie intake at our table increased noticeably. I continued to employ this strategy until it was enough a part of our dinner routine that we decided to name it the Veggie Course.

If my kids are hungry and I put pasta or rice on the table they will fill up on carbs and leave the veggies to the (very) last bite. Serving veggies first short-circuits that pattern. Bonus: It gives you extra time to prepare dinner. Artichokes remain our favorite Veggie Course dish. They are fun to eat, easy to share, and satisfying to hungry bellies (albeit, dipping their leaves in melted butter is a big part of the draw). But this strategy works with nearly any vegetable—sweet potato, kale, cauliflower, and rainbow carrots are the top candidates at our table—so take your pick.

Make It a Game: 15 points
Eat Your Colors: Green or Blue/Purple

> ### Invite Exploration
>
> "I wonder why artichokes are so tough on the outside?"
>
> "Do you think the size or color of the artichoke changes its flavor? Let's explore!"
>
> "Can you think of an easy way to remove the prickly core from an artichoke?"

Steamed Artichokes with Lemon Butter

The beauty of artichokes is that they are so simple to make, they look glamorous when they're done, and eating them is a tasty, fun adventure in itself! My kids enjoy peeling back the layers and noting how the texture changes as we get closer to the hidden treasure. The heart is the best part!

PREP TIME: 5 minutes

COOK TIME: 30 minutes

Serves 4

INGREDIENTS:

4 large artichokes

3 tablespoons unsalted butter

2 tablespoons lemon juice (from 1 lemon)

Cook Together

Beginners: Trim the leaves. Make the dressing.

Experts: Cut off the top rows and stem.

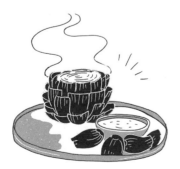

DIRECTIONS:

1   Using a pair of kitchen scissors, trim off a ½-inch section of the sharp ends of the artichoke leaves. Using a large serrated knife, cut off the top two rows of the artichoke, then the stem.

2   Place about 2 inches of water in a large saucepan. Bring to a boil.

3   Place the artichokes in a steamer basket, set it in the saucepan, and cover the pan. Steam the artichokes for 30 minutes, or until the leaves can be easily removed. Check the pot occasionally to make sure the water hasn't boiled away. (I learned this lesson the hard way after burning the bottom of a pot more than once!)

4   Remove the artichokes from the pan and let cool for 10 to 15 minutes.

5   While the artichokes are cooling, slowly melt the butter in a small saucepan over low heat or in the microwave for 30 seconds. Mix in the lemon juice.

6   Serve the sauce in individual dipping bowls alongside your freshly steamed artichokes.

Buy in Season When artichokes are in season, you'll find everything from miniature purple bundles to glorious green giants at your local market. Try a variety and compare tastes and textures.

Grilled Artichokes

Try grilling artichokes to experiment with taste and texture. This is another recipe that is one of my husband's specialties. In our house, Anthony is king of the grill. Try this recipe with Tasty Beef Skewers (page 284), another easy dish to make on the grill.

PREP TIME: 10 minutes

COOK TIME: 25 minutes

Serves 4

INGREDIENTS:

4 large artichokes

½ cup extra-virgin olive oil

¼ cup lemon juice (from about 2 lemons)

2 tablespoons finely chopped fresh mint

DIRECTIONS:

1 Using a pair of kitchen scissors, trim off a ½-inch section of the sharp ends of the artichoke leaves. Using a large serrated knife, cut off the top two rows of the artichokes, then the stem. Cut the artichokes into quarters and, using a melon baller, scoop out and discard the prickly choke.

2 Bring a large pot of water to a boil. Add the artichoke sections and boil for 15 minutes.

3 Drain the artichokes and let them cool. (This can be done the day before. Simply cover and refrigerate the artichokes if you're making them ahead.)

4 Heat a grill to medium-high heat. In a small bowl, whisk together the oil, lemon, and mint. Let your kids paint the artichokes with the dressing.

5 Grill the artichokes for about 10 minutes, or until they are lightly charred and the leaves can easily be removed. Drizzle some of the remaining dressing over the artichokes before serving, and reserve a bit in a small bowl for dipping.

Keep Trying Try lots of different combinations of vegetables for your Veggie Course, including artichokes. Experiment with familiar favorites along with new foods that your kids pick. Serving your veggies with a dip, like Nut-Free Basil Pesto (page 230), Greek Yogurt Dip (page 82), or Healthy Homemade Hummus (page 278), can help as well.

Brussels Sprouts

In the early days of feeding my family, I was notorious for making special meals for special people. But making a separate meal for my kids was contributing to battles at our family table. I realized it was a problem, so I looked for a simple place to start to make a change. I decided that Brussels sprouts, the most unlikely of vegetables, would be my antidote to the standard kids' menu of baby carrots and steamed broccoli.

In late November, our local market provided me with the perfect opening move. Thick, tall stalks studded with oversize green marbles were eye-catching—seeing Brussels sprouts in their native form was a big part of the allure, for all of us. Prying them from the stem and chopping them up was great fun, but in this case it was the sizzling of bacon that kept everyone on their toes, waiting for the first taste. Many adults, no less kids, find Brussels sprouts to be too bitter to stomach, so my expectations were low.

To my wonderful surprise, everyone enjoyed Brussels sprouts (including me). Whether it was because of their traditional association with holiday dinners, or because I felt the joy of everyone eating a meal without modifications, Brussels sprouts brought a festive feel to our regular weeknight dinner. They continue to show up on our family menu when fall brings them knocking.

Make It a Game: 15 points
Eat Your Colors: Green or Purple

Invite Exploration

"I wonder why Brussels sprouts grow on a stalk?"

"I wonder if Brussels sprouts taste different depending on their color?"

Roasted Brussels Sprouts

Brussels sprouts are one of my husband Anthony's favorite foods. He is masterful at making them. This dish is now firmly seated on our family favorites list. No kids' menu required.

PREP TIME: 10 minutes

COOK TIME: 20 to 25 minutes

Serves 4

INGREDIENTS:

1 pound Brussels sprouts, trimmed

4 slices thick bacon

1 tablespoon extra-virgin olive oil

¼ teaspoon kosher salt

Cook Together

Beginners: Pry the sprouts from the stalk.

Experts: Chop the sprouts.

DIRECTIONS:

1 Preheat the oven to 400°F.

2 Cut the sprouts in half lengthwise and place them on a rimmed baking sheet. If the heads are larger, cut them into quarters.

3 Cut the bacon into ½-inch pieces and add them to the sprouts. Use a pair of kitchen scissors to make cutting the bacon easier. (Parents should do this step.)

4 Drizzle the oil over the sprouts and bacon, sprinkle with salt, and toss to coat evenly. Spread the mixture in a single, even layer on the pan, arranging the cut sprouts flat side down.

5 Bake for 20 to 25 minutes, turning them once at the halfway point. You'll know the sprouts are ready when they're tender and crispy on the edges and the bacon is cooked through.

Tip *Chop everything in advance, toss it on a rimmed baking sheet, and cover with aluminum foil to save time during the dinner hustle.*

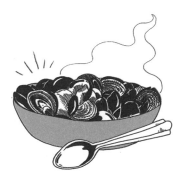

Brussels Sprouts Chips

Catherine's love of the crispy, almost burnt leaves of Roasted Brussels Sprouts (page 76) was our inspiration for Brussels Sprouts Chips—a riff on Kale Chips. This recipe takes some patience to prep but the result is well worth it. We especially love these chips paired with Anthony's Famous Short Ribs (page 285).

PREP TIME: 30 minutes

COOK TIME: 25 minutes

Serves 4

INGREDIENTS:

1 pound Brussels sprouts, trimmed

2 tablespoons extra-virgin olive oil

¼ teaspoon kosher salt

Cook Together

Beginners: Peel the leaves.

Experts: Cut away the ends.

DIRECTIONS:

1 Preheat the oven to 350°F.

2 Using your fingers, peel away the leaves from the sprouts.

3 Place the leaves on a rimmed baking sheet. Add the oil and salt and toss to combine.

4 Bake for 10 minutes, then toss the leaves in the pan. Reduce the heat to 250°F and bake the sprouts for 15 minutes more, or until the leaves are crispy and almost burnt. Let your kids watch closely to figure out the best timing for your oven.

Tip The easiest way to peel the leaves is to cut off the ends, turn the sprouts over and gently pry the leaves away starting at the stem. Keep trimming off the ends as you go to make it easier to peel off the layers. This takes patience (and time), but it's a fun activity for your kids. As you get closer to the center, the leaves will become too tight to peel, so simply save the small pieces for sautéing or roasting.

Keep Trying Catherine's preference for crispy leaves inspired us to try Brussels sprouts as chips. We followed her lead and discovered something new.

Buy in Season The best time to enjoy Brussels sprouts is during their short season in the late fall, around the holidays. To pick the perfect bunch, look for small, tight heads with no yellow or brown leaves. Seek them out, on the stalk, at your local market.

Sautéed Brussels Sprouts with Lemon and Walnuts

Paired with lemon and walnuts, this Brussels sprouts "slaw" provides a slightly different texture (and taste) to try with your kids.

PREP TIME: 10 minutes

COOK TIME: 8 minutes

Serves 4

INGREDIENTS:

1 pound Brussels sprouts, trimmed

2 tablespoons unsalted butter

1 tablespoon fresh lemon juice (from ½ lemon)

¼ cup coarsely chopped walnuts

¼ teaspoon kosher salt

DIRECTIONS:

1 Cut the sprouts in half lengthwise. With the flat side down, slice each half crosswise into 3 to 4 smaller sections and separate the leaves. Discard the ends.

2 In a large sauté pan, melt the butter over medium heat. Add the sprouts and sauté for 7 to 8 minutes, or until lightly browned and tender.

3 Transfer the cooked sprouts to a large serving bowl and combine with the lemon juice, walnuts, and salt.

4 Serve immediately.

Cook Together

To easily chop the walnuts, place them in a small plastic bag, then let your kids smash them with a rolling pin.

Keep Trying

The bitterness of Brussels sprouts will vary depending on how they are prepared. Try them roasted and sautéed to find the right flavor for your kids.

Fun at the Family Table: (Word) Play with Your Food

After a long day, it's often hard to spark a conversation at your family table beyond the typical one-word answers to common questions like, "How was your day?" Simple games are an easy way to get everyone engaged and talking.

A word study in James' class uncovered another way to play with food. Inspired by an investigation of words and their meanings, we started a hunt for homophones (words that sound the same but have different meanings). At each dinner, we build onto our list of "food" words that play tricks. Try it with your kids, and add to the list.

Homophones
Words that have the same sound, but different spelling and meaning.

> Beet (the vegetable) and Beat (a rhythmic unit in music)
> Chews (to bite food) and Choose (to pick something from a selection of alternatives)
> Palate (a person's experience of taste) and Palette (a board used by an artist to mix paint)
> Flour (an ingredient made from wheat) and Flower (a plant in our garden)

Homographs
Words that have the same spelling but a different meaning. In some cases, they are pronounced differently.

> Mint (an herb that grows in your garden versus the place where they make money)
> Buffet (a type of table versus to strike)
> Bass (a type of fish versus a kind of string instrument)
> Minute (a unit of time versus a very small amount of something)

A special note of thanks to my son James' teachers, Emily Mitchell and Sam Modest, for inspiring this never-ending search for the meaning of words at our family table. And to Pete Bowers, for helping it all make sense.

Cauliflower

When Catherine announced that she liked tasting cauliflower from the school garden, I enthusiastically started working white, orange, and purple cauliflower into our weekly menu. I roasted a big batch of cauliflower to a beautiful golden, crispy brown. I thought she would love it. But she didn't.

"You said you loved cauliflower!" I said, the temperature in my voice rising.

"I do like cauliflower," Catherine offered, "but I prefer it raw."

Well, I hadn't thought of that! I cringe at the sight (or smell or taste) of raw cauliflower. But that's exactly the point. It wasn't about me. It was about Catherine—her preferences, her experience of tastes and textures, and her ability to figure out what works for her and to choose for herself.

Catherine's preference for raw cauliflower opened up some unexpected opportunities. The perfect complement to raw veggies is a healthy dip, so we spent a few weeks experimenting with dressings to pair with our new pal cauliflower. Our biggest successes were with a healthy Greek Yogurt Dip (page 82), kind of like tzatziki but milder, Healthy Homemade Hummus (page 278), and James' favorite, Nut-Free Basil Pesto (page 230). Speaking of James, he prefers his cauliflower roasted, like I do. The crispier (and more colorful) the better.

So now when we make cauliflower, we wash and prepare it together, and then set aside a bowl of raw rosettes with a dip, and roast up the rest. It's an easy way to let everyone have it their way while we enjoy the pleasure of eating the same food.

Make It a Game: 10 points
Eat Your Colors: White, Yellow/Orange, Blue/Purple

Invite Exploration

"Can you measure 3 cups of cauliflower using each measuring cup only once?"

Roasted Purple Cauliflower

Roasting cauliflower is an easy weeknight side dish. Try this recipe with a combination of purple, yellow, and white cauliflower for an easy way to add more colors to your table.

PREP TIME: 10 minutes

COOK TIME: 20 minutes

Serves 4

INGREDIENTS:

1 head purple cauliflower, cut into ½-inch pieces

1 tablespoon extra-virgin olive oil

¼ teaspoon kosher salt

1 tablespoon fresh lemon juice (from ½ lemon)

DIRECTIONS:

1 Preheat the oven to 400°F.

2 On a rimmed baking sheet, toss the cauliflower with the oil and salt.

3 Roast for 20 minutes, turning once, until the edges of the cauliflower are brown and crispy.

4 Before serving, add the lemon juice and toss to coat.

Tip To easily chop cauliflower, turn the head upside down and use a paring knife to cut around the core to remove it. Then, chop the larger florets into bite-size pieces.

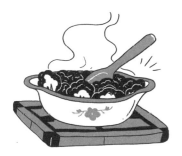

Cook Together

Beginners: Using your hands, break apart the cauliflower into smaller florets.

Experts: Cut the cauliflower.

Greek Yogurt Dip

An easy dip that I like to pair with raw cauliflower and other fresh veggies is made with Greek yogurt and lemon juice. You can also try Nut-Free Basil Pesto (page 230) or Healthy Homemade Hummus (page 278).

PREP TIME: 5 minutes

COOK TIME: 0 minutes

Makes ½ cup

INGREDIENTS:

⅓ cup nonfat plain Greek yogurt

3 tablespoons extra-virgin olive oil

2 tablespoons grated Parmesan cheese

1 tablespoon fresh lemon juice (from ½ lemon)

1 garlic clove, finely chopped, or 1 clove Roasted Garlic (page 69)

¼ teaspoon kosher salt

DIRECTIONS:

1 In a food processor, combine the yogurt, oil, Parmesan, lemon juice, garlic, and salt. Process for 2 to 3 minutes, or until the mixture is smooth and consistent.

2 Transfer to a glass container and store in the refrigerator for up to 1 week.

Keep Trying Try cauliflower raw, roasted, and sautéed. Serve it with a dip and without. Compare.

Rainbow Carrots

At the height of our mealtime battles, it was challenging to get one vegetable onto the table, much less two (or three). Most nights, I considered myself lucky if peas made it onto the menu. But as we started focusing on boosting colors on our plates, I needed to find simple ways to get more vegetables on the table, and ones that didn't require much cooking. Rainbow carrots were an easy solution—three colors in one.

Like artichokes, I served sliced rainbow carrots (with or without a dip) before the start of our meal as an easy way to get the veggies in first. I found that I could manage to make one cooked side dish, like Crispy Kale Chips (page 124) or Roasted Purple Cauliflower (page 81), but making two recipes was often a challenge, especially on weeknights. Instead, I would offer raw rainbow carrots to round out our colors without much added work.

Beyond ease of preparation, these little powerhouses are packed with vitamins, and each color plays a role—orange delivers vitamin A, red provides lycopene, and purple is packed with anthocyanins.[5] The easiest way to feature them at your table is cut into sticks and paired with a dip like Healthy Homemade Hummus (page 278) or sliced thin like ribbons and tossed with lemon juice. Cooking them increases their benefits even further, releasing more of those powerful antioxidants.[6] Try them roasted like fries, or use them as a variation in Magic Leaf Soup (page 98) or Power Lunch Veggie Stir-Fry (page 141).

Make It a Game: 10 points
Eat Your Colors: Red, Yellow/Orange, Blue/Purple, White

Invite Exploration

"What do you think gives rainbow carrots their color?"

Roasted Rainbow Carrot Sticks

Roasting carrots is an easy variation on this workhorse vegetable, plus it releases even more of the nutrients packed inside. Bonus!

PREP TIME: 10 minutes

COOK TIME: 20 minutes

Serves 4

INGREDIENTS:

2 bunches rainbow carrots
(12 to 16 medium carrots)

2 tablespoons extra-virgin
olive oil

½ teaspoon kosher salt

DIRECTIONS:

1   Preheat the oven to 400°F.

2   Wash and cut the carrots into 3-inch-long sections, then cut each section into equal-size sticks.

3   Place the carrots on a rimmed baking sheet, then add the oil and salt. Toss to coat thoroughly. Arrange them in a single, even layer on the pan.

4   Roast the carrots for 10 minutes. Flip them, then continue to bake for 10 minutes more, or until the carrots are slightly caramelized and brown on the edges.

Cook Together

The healthy nutrients in rainbow carrots live close to the surface. Instead of peeling all of that goodness away, just give them a good scrub. If you choose to peel, do so lightly.

Grow It   Carrots are relatively easy to grow. They will tolerate cooler temperatures, so you can start in early spring—a few weeks before the last frost.

Rainbow Ribbons

This is an easy alternative to sliced raw carrots. The lemon juice and mint give this dish a refreshing flavor.

PREP TIME: 10 minutes

WAIT TIME: 15 minutes

Serves 4

INGREDIENTS:

1 bunch rainbow carrots
(6 to 8 carrots)

1 tablespoon fresh lemon juice
(from ½ lemon)

1 tablespoon coarsely chopped
fresh mint

¼ teaspoon kosher salt

DIRECTIONS:

1 Wash the carrots, and using a vegetable peeler, shave the carrots into long, thin layers.

2 In a large bowl, combine the carrots with the lemon juice, oil, mint, and salt. Cover and place in the refrigerator for 15 minutes to let the flavors meld before serving.

Tip *For an easy variation, add thinly shaved fennel or parsnips to the carrots.*

Cook Together

Shaving carrots can be tricky for some kids. To make it easier, cut the carrots in half through the middle. Place flat side down on a cutting board and then peel into long, thin layers. Be sure to shave the carrots *away* from yourself. When they get whittled down, simply cut them into sticks and serve on the side with a dip.

Cook with Friends

Standing on our front doorstep with outstretched arms was Catherine's friend Mari. She had just arrived for an afternoon of fun and was showing us her contribution.

"I brought rainbow carrots. I chose them because they are really good in soups and the colors were so pretty. I found them at the farmers' market."

Inspired by a recipe challenge issued by First Lady Michelle Obama, my daughter, Catherine, had invited three of her closest friends to a cooking playdate. The invitation to each child was simple: Bring a favorite vegetable from your garden or the farmers' market and join us for an afternoon of cooking "Friendship Garden Soup."

When I asked what inspired her idea, Catherine explained, "My idea for Friendship Garden Soup came from a book I read when I was little. The book is called *Stone Soup* and tells the story of villagers who bring food to make a soup with a stone in it. They learned to make something special by sharing everything they had. So I thought that it would be nice to invite my friends to share vegetables from their own gardens. When you share it makes everything better."

In a garden get-together worthy of the classic tale, my daughter and her friends spent the afternoon cooking together. Like wizards, they gathered around the simmering pot and theorized about which ingredients they should add to maximize its power. They packed it with colors: red and orange carrots, green peas and celery, white and purple cauliflower.

The best part of this activity was how a community of friends came together to create something special. Each child contributed something different to add to the soup's unique flavor, in the same way that each friend brings something unique and special to my daughter's life.

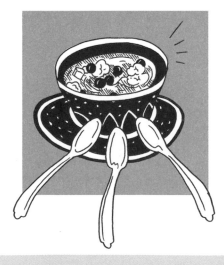

Friendship Garden Soup

Invite friends to bring any vegetable that they like from their garden or the local farmers' market, and enjoy an afternoon cooking together.

PREP TIME: 30 minutes

COOK TIME: 25 to 30 minutes

Serves 6

INGREDIENTS:

1 tablespoon extra-virgin olive oil

½ medium onion, diced

4 carrots, cut into ½-inch pieces (about 1 cup)

2 stalks celery, cut into ½-inch pieces (about 1 cup)

½ head cauliflower, cut into ½-inch pieces (about 1 cup)

8 cups Chicken Broth (page 99)

1 cup Easy Roasted Chicken (page 282), cut into ½-inch cubes

1 handful fresh oregano leaves

1 bay leaf

1 cup uncooked pasta (macaroni or rotini work best)

1 cup fresh English peas, shelled

Kosher salt and freshly ground black pepper

DIRECTIONS:

1 Heat a large stockpot over medium heat. Add the oil and onion and sauté for 2 to 3 minutes, or until the onions are soft and fragrant.

2 Add the carrots, celery, and cauliflower and cook, stirring occasionally, for about 5 minutes, or until the veggies are slightly browned.

3 Add the broth, chicken, oregano, and bay leaf. Cover and bring to a boil. Add the pasta, then reduce the heat to maintain a simmer and cook for 10 minutes, or until the vegetables begin to soften and the pasta is cooked through.

4 Add the fresh peas and simmer for 1 minute more.

5 Season with salt and pepper to taste before serving.

Tip You can add almost any vegetable to this recipe, which makes it forgiving. Just be sure to put in onion, celery, and carrots—they form the base of the soup.

Cook Together

Beginners: Harvest the vegetables or source them from the farmers' market. Remove peas from the pods. Stir the pot.

Experts: Dice the vegetables.

Pumpkin

When my kids were in preschool, the class would attempt to grow a pumpkin each year, most times with success. To watch that tiny seed emerge as a big, happy orange ball was incredibly rewarding for my kids. When the school harvest was slim, nearby farms would offer ample supply. In October, there never seems to be a shortage of pumpkins!

Carving pumpkins of all shapes and sizes into a family of jack-o'-lanterns is an autumn activity we treasure. Like gingerbread houses at Christmas, it marks the season. But beyond the fun of Halloween, pumpkins provide volumes of wonderful, easy recipes to cook together, and a great example of how to use the whole plant.

Last fall, Catherine hosted a cooking class at school. Her goal: Use the whole pumpkin. First came the seeds. Scooping out those little gourds was messy, but the kind of fun that Catherine loves. Roasted pumpkin seeds provided a welcome late-afternoon snack for her classmates and left them longing for the next dish. The following week, we roasted the pumpkins to make puree that we transformed into pie, bread, and soup. The skins made their way to the garden compost, to complete the cycle.

I used to think it was simply easier to buy premade pumpkin puree. No arguing that it's easier, but the rewards of roasting your own are much greater, if only to feel the satisfaction of using the whole plant.

Make It a Game: 15 points

Eat Your Colors: Yellow/Orange

Invite Exploration

"How would you get the seeds out of the pumpkin?"

"I wonder if the color on the inside of a pumpkin changes depending on the skin color?"

Savory or Spiced Roasted Pumpkin Seeds

Roasting pumpkin seeds is a fun family cooking project and a great way to show your kids how to enjoy the whole plant. Plus, a big batch of freshly roasted pumpkin seeds makes an easy Halloween treat or lunchbox snack.

PREP TIME: 15 minutes

COOK TIME: 15 to 20 minutes

Serves 4

INGREDIENTS:

1 medium sugar pumpkin

1 tablespoon extra-virgin olive oil

¼ teaspoon kosher salt

Ground cinnamon (optional)

Ground nutmeg (optional)

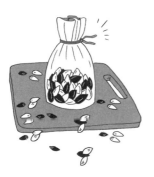

DIRECTIONS:

1   Preheat the oven to 350°F.

2   Cut the pumpkin in half lengthwise. Using a melon baller or a spoon, scoop out the seeds and stringy insides of the pumpkin and place them in a large bowl. Reserve the pumpkin to make Pumpkin Puree (page 90).

3   Fill the bowl with water. The seeds will float to the top. Using your fingers, release any seeds that remain caught in the flesh of the pumpkin. Remove any large chunks of flesh and place them in the compost. Skim across the top of the water with your hands to capture and remove the seeds and place them in a sieve. Wash and drain the seeds, removing any remaining flesh.

4   In a small saucepan, bring 2 cups water to a boil. Add the seeds and boil gently for 10 minutes, then drain the seeds in a sieve. This extra step makes for extra-plump and crispy seeds.

Tip Choose one pumpkin for each person, so everyone can scoop their own. Smaller pumpkins, like the sugar variety, are easier for little hands to handle and are also better for cooking. This is a messy job! Set up your project outside, if possible, so you can give your kids plenty of space to master their scooping technique.

Cook Together

Beginners: Scoop out and separate the seeds. Season the seeds.

Experts: Slice the pumpkin.

5 Transfer the seeds to a rimmed baking sheet and toss them with the oil. Spread the seeds into a single, even layer on the pan.

6 Bake, stirring occasionally, for 15 to 20 minutes, or until the seeds turn golden brown and begin to pop.

7 Set the baking sheet on a wire rack and let the seeds cool completely.

8 In a medium bowl, toss the seeds with the salt for a savory treat. For a spiced treat, add a dash of cinnamon and nutmeg.

Pumpkin Puree

It may be easier to buy pumpkin puree in a can, but the flavor of fresh roasted pumpkin just can't be beat, in my opinion. It's super easy to make, and a fun cooking project for your kids. Make the puree ahead and store it in a glass container in your fridge. Work it into fall treats like Homemade Pumpkin Pie with Gingersnap Crust (page 91) or Pumpkin Bread (page 92).

PREP TIME: 10 minutes
COOK TIME: 60 minutes
Makes 2 to 3 cups

INGREDIENTS:
1 medium sugar pumpkin
(2 to 3 pounds)

Grow It
Pumpkins need plenty of space to grow. Wait for late spring, then plant in a sunny location. If you're lucky, your great pumpkin will appear in early fall.

DIRECTIONS:

1 Preheat the oven to 350°F. Line a rimmed baking sheet with foil or parchment paper.

2 Cut the pumpkin in half lengthwise. Using a melon baller or spoon, scoop out the seeds and stringy core, then cut out the stem. Reserve the seeds to make Savory or Spiced Roasted Pumpkin Seeds (pages 89–90).

3 Place the pumpkin facedown on the lined baking sheet. Bake for 60 minutes, or until the skin is brown and slightly charred and the flesh is tender when pierced with a fork.

4 Let cool, then using a large spoon, scoop the pulp into a bowl. Run the pulp through a food mill, or mash with a potato masher, to create a smooth puree.

5 Cover and refrigerate for up to 1 week. The puree can also be frozen for up to 1 month.

Homemade Pumpkin Pie with Gingersnap Crust

This recipe is a variation on my gram's old-fashioned pumpkin pie. She used to make it with canned pumpkin, but it's even better with homemade Pumpkin Puree (page 90). Use a premade crust (with natural ingredients you can identify) if you don't have time to make your own.

PREP TIME: 20 minutes

COOK TIME: 65 minutes

Serves 12

INGREDIENTS:

FOR THE CRUST:

3 cups gingersnap cookies

¼ cup light brown sugar

1 tablespoon whole wheat all-purpose flour

½ teaspoon kosher salt

4 tablespoons (½ stick) unsalted butter, melted

FOR THE FILLING:

½ cup light brown sugar

1 teaspoon ground cinnamon

¾ teaspoon ground ginger

¼ teaspoon ground cloves

½ teaspoon kosher salt

2 cups Pumpkin Puree (page 90)

3 large eggs, beaten

¾ cup nonfat milk

Vanilla ice cream or whipped cream, for serving

DIRECTIONS:

FOR THE CRUST:

1 Preheat the oven to 350°F.

2 Using a food processor, process the gingersnap cookies into crumbs. You should have about 1¾ cups of crumbs.

3 Transfer the crumbs to a large bowl and whisk in the sugar, flour, and salt. Add the melted butter to the gingersnap mixture and stir well. The mixture should stick together when pressed with your fingers. If not, add up to 1 tablespoon cold water.

4 Press the crumb mixture into the bottom and up the sides of a 9-inch pie plate. Bake for 10 minutes, or until golden brown.

5 Let cool completely before filling with the pumpkin mixture.

FOR THE FILLING:

1 Increase the oven temperature to 425°F.

2 In a large bowl, combine the sugar, cinnamon, ginger, cloves, and salt.

3 Add the pumpkin puree, eggs, and milk and stir gently to combine.

4 Pour the pumpkin mixture into the gingersnap crust and bake for 10 minutes. Reduce the heat to 350°F and bake for 45 minutes more, or until a knife inserted into the filling comes out clean. Remove from the oven and let cool completely on a wire rack.

5 Serve with vanilla ice cream or whipped cream.

Pumpkin Bread

Pumpkin bread is another easy recipe to make with your pumpkin puree. It's equally great served at breakfast or in your kids' lunchboxes.

PREP TIME: 15 minutes

COOK TIME: 20 minutes

Serves 8

INGREDIENTS:

2 large eggs, beaten

½ cup light brown sugar

1 cup Pumpkin Puree (page 90)

¼ cup grapeseed oil

¼ cup nonfat plain yogurt

1½ cups whole wheat all-purpose flour

1 teaspoon ground cinnamon

1 teaspoon baking soda

1 teaspoon baking powder

½ teaspoon ground ginger

½ teaspoon kosher salt

Confectioners' sugar, for dusting

DIRECTIONS:

1 Preheat the oven to 350°F. Spray a 9 x 9-inch cake pan with olive oil.

2 In the bowl of a stand mixer fitted with the whisk attachment, combine the eggs and the brown sugar. Beat on high speed for 2 to 3 minutes or until fluffy. Add the pumpkin puree, oil, and yogurt. Mix on medium speed for 2 to 3 minutes, or until the mixture is fully combined.

3 In a separate bowl, whisk together the flour, cinnamon, baking soda, baking powder, ginger, and salt.

4 Working in small batches, add the flour mixture to the pumpkin mixture. Stir gently to combine.

5 Pour the batter into the prepared pan and bake for 20 minutes, or until the top is golden brown and springs back when lightly touched. A toothpick inserted into the center of the loaf should come out clean. Cool in the pan for 10 minutes, then transfer the loaf to a wire rack to cool completely.

6 Sprinkle with a dusting of confectioners' sugar before serving.

Tip *Add 1 cup of fresh whole cranberries for extra color.*

Buy in Season A visit to the local pumpkin patch is one of our favorite fall activities. Ask the farmer which types of pumpkins and gourds grow on their farm, and how you can tell the difference between each variety.

Butternut Squash

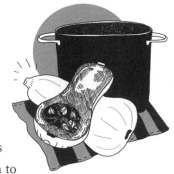

Butternut squash soup—the one that came in the little orange box with the easy pour spout—was a dish that I served each year at Thanksgiving. Before we started our 52 New Foods Challenge, I hadn't given much thought to this dish other than to remember to keep it stacked in our pantry at holiday time. But as we grew more comfortable in our new-food environment, slowly shifting our purchases from the grocery store to the farmers' market, I found that I grew out of the need (or desire) for boxed soup.

Instead of buying butternut squash soup, I decided to learn how to make it from scratch. It turned out to be another fun cooking project with my kids—scooping out the seeds was much like our adventure with pumpkin, and roasting the gourd made the whole house smell wonderful. Making our own soup was more work, and it definitely took more time, but the flavor was so much better. And because my kids had a hand in making our soup, they were willing to give it a taste, which was a step in the right direction.

On a busy parent's schedule, I know it's hard to reduce your reliance on boxes, bags, and cans. So start with one food to make from scratch, like soup. Try it at holiday time—it's easy to make ahead. Cut yourself some slack and use boxed organic chicken broth, but all fresh ingredients. When you're ready for more, prepare your own Chicken Broth (page 99). Work up to making a simple, homemade soup once a month. Freeze a portion each time so you start to build up some reserves. You'll find that it's easier than you think once you get into the rhythm.

Make It a Game: 15 points
Eat Your Colors: Yellow/Orange

> **Invite Exploration**
>
> "What do you notice that's similar about pumpkins and butternut squash?"

Butternut Squash Puree

This delicious puree is one of my favorite bases for fall soups. Try it as the feature in Easy Butternut Squash Soup (page 95) or blend it gently into Magic Leaf Soup (page 98) to give the soup a creamy texture. This recipe can be made ahead, and stored in a glass container in your fridge, to save you time.

PREP TIME: 10 minutes

COOK TIME: 30 minutes

Makes about 3 cups

INGREDIENTS:

1 large butternut squash
(about 3 pounds)

DIRECTIONS:

1 Preheat the oven to 400°F. Line a rimmed baking sheet with a Silpat mat.

2 Cut the squash in half lengthwise. Scoop out and discard the seeds.

3 Place the squash facedown on the lined baking sheet.

4 Bake for 30 minutes, or until the flesh can be easily scooped out with a spoon.

5 Let cool, then scoop the flesh into a bowl. Run the squash through a food mill or mash with a potato masher to make a puree. The puree can be stored in the refrigerator for up to 1 week or frozen for up to 1 month.

Easy Butternut Squash Soup

My kids loved how the smell of this simple soup brought back fond memories of family celebrations. It also freezes well, so make extra for your reserves.

PREP TIME: 30 minutes

COOK TIME: 25 minutes

Serves 6 to 8

INGREDIENTS:

2 tablespoons extra-virgin olive oil

1 small onion, chopped

2 cups Butternut Squash Puree (page 94)

2 cups Chicken Broth (page 99)

Kosher salt, to taste

Fresh parsley, for garnish

DIRECTIONS:

1 Heat a medium stockpot over medium heat. Add the oil and onions and simmer gently for 2 to 3 minutes, or until the onions are soft and fragrant.

2 Add the squash puree and broth to the onions. Cover, bring to a boil, then reduce the heat to low and simmer for 20 minutes.

3 Let the butternut squash mixture cool slightly, then carefully transfer it to a blender and blend for 2 minutes or until smooth. (Be careful when pureeing hot liquids.)

4 Transfer the soup back to the pot and warm it gently before serving. Season with kosher salt to taste. Garnish with fresh parsley.

Cook Together

Beginners: Scoop out the seeds. Scoop out the roasted flesh. Stir the soup.

Experts: Slice the squash. Chop the squash.

Tip: A melon baller makes it easier for kids to scoop out the seeds.

Keep Trying

Butternut Squash Puree (page 94) can be used in lots of different ways. Add it to any homemade soup to give it a creamy flavor. Blend it into mac 'n' cheese, but don't hide it. No sneaking! Be sure to have your kids mix it in so they know what's in their food.

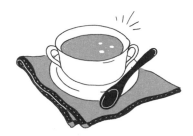

Maple-Roasted Butternut Squash

Another easy way to prepare butternut squash is to simply peel and roast it. A touch of maple syrup makes this recipe even more delicious.

PREP TIME: 10 minutes

COOK TIME: 30 minutes

Serves 6

INGREDIENTS:

1 large butternut squash
(about 3 pounds)

2 tablespoons extra-virgin
olive oil

2 tablespoons pure maple
syrup

½ teaspoon kosher salt

Grow It Plant your squash along with your pumpkin in late spring.

DIRECTIONS:

1 Preheat the oven to 400°F.

2 Peel the squash. Cut it in half lengthwise and scoop out and discard the seeds. Chop the squash into large cubes, about 1 inch.

3 On a rimmed baking sheet, combine the squash, oil, maple syrup, and salt. Spread the squash in a single, even layer on the pan.

4 Bake, turning once, for 25 to 30 minutes, or until the squash is brown on the edges and tender when pierced with a fork.

Make It a Main

While the squash is roasting, follow the directions for Okra Risotto (page 259), substituting the Maple-Roasted Butternut Squash for the chopped okra.

The worst offender in our pantry was canned chicken noodle soup. For all of the fresh food we had been eating, those cans of soup stuck out like a sore thumb. I have no idea why I kept hanging on to them. Maybe tradition? For my husband and me, canned chicken noodle soup was a childhood staple. What else would we serve when someone had the sniffles?

Those sniffles were what prompted a reevaluation. James woke early one winter morning with a terrible fever—the kind of soaring temperature that makes me want to sleep next to him to keep a close watch. I stumbled down to the kitchen to start the soup, reached into the pantry to grab a can, then paused. I just couldn't do a heat-and-eat.

"I need to make it from scratch," I resolved. My husband, the sweetheart that he is, headed out to the market at the crack of dawn with a simple list—carrots, celery, and an onion. I had some leftover chicken in the fridge from dinner the previous night.

"Why does chicken soup help to make me feel better when I am sick?" James asked. This question is one I've asked myself many times over.

"I'm not sure," I replied. "Why do you think it helps?"

His little hands wrapped around the bowl, sipping slowly, he pondered this question and then responded, "Maybe the vegetables chase the bugs away." I smiled a big smile and hugged him tight.

"You know, I think you may be right. I'm glad that you're feeling better."

As for the cans, I put them out to use as doorstops.

Magic Leaf Soup

My son, James, calls this recipe Magic Leaf Soup because his job is to add the bay leaf. He says it gives this soup its special flavor (and cold-fighting power).

PREP TIME: 15 minutes

COOK TIME: 15 minutes

Serves 6

INGREDIENTS:

3 stalks celery

2 carrots

DIRECTIONS:

1 Chop the celery, carrots, and onion into ¼- to ½-inch pieces. Finely mince the garlic, avoiding any large chunks.

2 Heat a large stockpot over medium heat. Add the oil, garlic, and onions and cook gently for 2 to 3 minutes, or until the onions are translucent. Add the carrots and celery

½ onion

1 clove garlic

1 tablespoon extra-virgin olive oil

4 cups Chicken Broth (below)

1 cup water

1 bay leaf

1 cup dry pasta (macaroni or rotini work best)

2 cups Simple Sautéed Chicken (page 283), chopped

Kosher salt and freshly ground black pepper

A few sprigs fresh thyme

and cook for 2 to 3 minutes more, or until the vegetables begin to soften.

3   Add the broth, 1 cup water, and the bay leaf. Cover and bring to a boil. Add the pasta, then reduce the heat to low and simmer for 8 minutes, or until the pasta is almost cooked.

4   Add the chicken to the pot and simmer for 2 minutes more.

5   Season to taste with salt and pepper. Serve warm, with a few sprigs of fresh thyme from your garden.

Chicken Broth

Whenever roast chicken is on our menu, my husband, Anthony, makes chicken broth. It's a great way to use the leftovers and yields a base for lots of recipes, including our favorite soups.

PREP TIME: 10 minutes

COOK TIME: 20 minutes

Makes 6 to 8 cups

INGREDIENTS:

1 tablespoon extra-virgin olive oil

1 medium onion, coarsely chopped

3 stalks celery, cut into ½-inch pieces

3 carrots, cut into ½-inch pieces

8 cups water

1 whole chicken carcass, cooked

1 bay leaf

1 teaspoon kosher salt

DIRECTIONS:

1   Heat a large stockpot over medium heat. Add the oil, onion, celery, and carrots and sauté for 2 to 3 minutes, or until the onions are soft and the carrots and celery are slightly browned.

2   Increase the heat to high. Add 8 cups water, then the chicken carcass, bay leaf, and salt. Cover and bring to a boil. Reduce the heat to low and simmer for 20 minutes.

3   Strain the broth through a sieve into a large bowl. Discard the bones. Save the meat and veggies for chicken soup. Cool the broth, then store it in a glass container in the refrigerator for up to 1 week. It can also be frozen for up to 1 month.

Apples

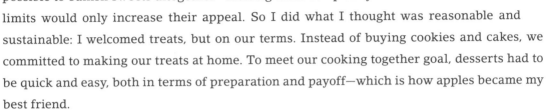

My weakness for treats is infamous. I have been known to
quickly power through a meal just to get to the sweet reward
at the end. Knowing this about myself, I decided it would be impossible to banish sweets altogether—making them completely off-
limits would only increase their appeal. So I did what I thought was reasonable and
sustainable: I welcomed treats, but on our terms. Instead of buying cookies and cakes, we
committed to making our treats at home. To meet our cooking together goal, desserts had to
be quick and easy, both in terms of preparation and payoff—which is how apples became my
best friend.

As one of nature's fast foods, apples can easily star as a seasonal dessert without any
preparation other than slicing. A colorful platter of sliced seasonal fruit—think yellow, red,
and green apples—is a fantastic dessert strategy and one that I'd recommend instituting on
weeknights to fend off too many sweet treats. But when the occasion calls for a little something more, apples can easily transform into something very special with minimal effort—a
warm bowl of cinnamon apples is an especially cozy treat, as is our personal favorite: Apple
Galette (page 101).

Apples may be a familiar food at your family table, but remember that they can help you
in myriad ways. Slice them up and offer them as an alternative to sugary desserts. Have fun
cooking them with your kids—they'll love all the peeling. And enjoy comparing the tastes
and textures of different apple varieties—there are so many to explore, together.

Make It a Game: 5 points
Eat Your Colors: Red, Yellow/Orange, Green

Invite Exploration

"What would make it easier to peel an apple?"

Apple Galette

This recipe is a simple rendition of an apple pie and is one of our favorite sweet treats. The beauty of this dish is that it doesn't have to be perfect to be delicious. It's a forgiving recipe, so let go and let your kids take the lead.

PREP TIME: 20 minutes

WAIT TIME: 45 minutes

COOK TIME: 60 minutes

Serves 6

INGREDIENTS:

2 pounds Braeburn apples

2 tablespoons fresh lemon juice (from 1 lemon)

1 teaspoon ground cinnamon

¼ cup plus 1 tablespoon light brown sugar

1 teaspoon pure vanilla extract

2 tablespoons unsalted butter

1 premade dessert pastry piecrust (12-inch diameter)

1 large egg

1 teaspoon nonfat milk

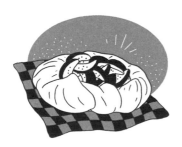

DIRECTIONS:

1   Line two rimmed baking sheets with parchment paper. Peel and cut the apples into wedges between ¼ and ½ inch wide.

2   In a large bowl, toss the apples with the lemon juice, cinnamon, ¼ cup of the sugar, and the vanilla.

3   In a large frying pan, melt the butter over medium heat. When the butter is bubbling (but before it turns brown), add the apple mixture. Toss gently in the pan. Cook for 5 to 7 minutes, or until the apples are brown on one side. Turn the apples gently to cook the other side. Simmer for 5 minutes more, or until the apples are golden brown and fragrant.

4   Place the cooked apples on one of the lined baking sheets and let cool.

5   Once the apples are cool, place the piecrust on the other lined baking sheet. If you're using a frozen crust, allow it to thaw slightly before using (about 10 minutes). Pile the apples in the center of the crust, then fold the pastry around the edges of your pie. Don't worry about perfect pleats! Let go and let your kids do the folding, leaving a little window in the center for the apples to peer through. Place the galette in the freezer for 45 minutes. This will help it to keep its shape when baked.

6   Preheat the oven to 350°F.

7   Remove the galette from the freezer. Beat the egg together with the milk to create an egg wash and let your kids paint the edges of the galette. Sprinkle with the remaining 1 tablespoon sugar.

Tip *When I have the time, I love to make my own piecrust. But with busy schedules in full swing, I often need an easier solution: premade pastry crust. If you go this route, be sure to pick a crust that has five ingredients or less. The ingredient list on the one that I use is simple: unbleached organic flour, butter, water, and salt.*

8 Bake for 1 hour, or until the edges are crispy and the apple mixture is bubbling.

9 Serve warm or cool, whichever you prefer.

Recipe inspired by Martha Rose Shulman of the New York Times.

Cook Together

Beginners: Peel the apples. Arrange the fruit. Pleat the edges of the piecrust. Paint the edges with the egg wash.

Experts: Cut the apples.

Tip: My kids find it easiest to use a potato peeler to remove the skins of an apple. Don't worry about being perfect! Even if the apples brown (because your kids are working slowly) they will ultimately taste delicious when you cook them.

Warm Cinnamon Apples

These cinnamon apples taste like the best part of an apple pie—the filling! They are delicious tucked into our Healthy Crepes (page 117) or served in small ramekins with (or without) scoops of vanilla ice cream.

PREP TIME: 10 minutes

COOK TIME: 10 minutes

Serves 4

INGREDIENTS:

4 large McIntosh apples (Granny Smiths are great, too)

¼ cup light brown sugar

½ teaspoon ground cinnamon

2 tablespoons fresh lemon juice (from 1 lemon)

1 tablespoon unsalted butter

Vanilla ice cream, for serving

DIRECTIONS:

1 Peel the apples and cut into ½-inch wedges.

2 In a medium bowl, combine the apples with the sugar, cinnamon, and lemon juice.

3 In a large frying pan, melt the butter over medium heat until bubbling but not brown. Add the apple mixture and cook, turning once, for 8 to 10 minutes, or until the apples are tender and brown on the edges.

4 Serve warm, with scoops of vanilla ice cream.

Buy in Season Ask your local farmer to point out unique varieties of apples and how they compare in terms of taste and texture.

Apple Chips

These crunchy chips make a great lunchbox snack. They take a while to bake, but they are worth it. Keep a big batch of these chips in a glass jar in your pantry to make them easy for you and your kids to grab when hunger strikes!

PREP TIME: 5 minutes

COOK TIME: 90 minutes

Serves 4

INGREDIENTS:

4 large Granny Smith apples

DIRECTIONS:

1   Preheat the oven to 250°F. Line two rimmed baking sheets with aluminum foil and spray lightly with olive oil (or line them with a Silpat mat, no oil required).

2   Leaving the skin on, slice the apples crosswise into thin layers, about ¼ inch thick. Remove the seeds. Note the pattern, and the Fibonacci sequence (see page 138), inside.

3   Divide the slices evenly between the baking sheets and bake for 60 minutes. Flip the apples, then bake for 30 minutes more, or until the slices are light brown and crispy. Thicker slices will be a little more chewy. For extra-crispy chips, leave the apples in the oven 15 minutes more. Timing will depend on the moisture content in your apples.

4   Let the chips cool completely, then store in your pantry in an airtight container for up to 1 week.

Cook Together

Slicing the apples in this recipe can be tricky and is best done by an adult. Cut a small section off the side of the fruit to make a flat base. Stand the fruit on the flat base, then cut. Invite your kids to arrange the slices on the rimmed baking sheets.

Pears

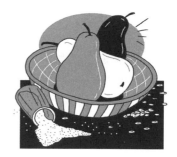

When pears are in season, I gobble them up like they are never going to be grown again. The textures of pears run the full gamut—from mouthwateringly soft to crisp and crunchy. They are one of my favorite sweet treats in the fall. When they arrive at the market, I fill our basket with every wonderful variety, working our way through the alphabet—Anjou, Bosc, Comice. James loves pears, too; Catherine's preference is still for apples. But we had a way to win her over: fruit crisps.

Not only are fruit crisps a gentle way to work in the flavor of new food, they are a great place to start when you're learning to cook with your kids—full of fruit (albeit with a sinfully delicious topping), fun to make, and flexible. It's pretty hard to mess up a fruit crisp. The whole point is to make them look messy in the first place!

Enjoying the no-pressure pleasure of making something delicious together, and the warm, cuddly embrace of a perfect pear crisp, paired with a few tart apples for good measure, was enough to convince Catherine to give pears a try. More than anything else, though, it was the experience of cooking together that had a bigger impact on us (especially me) than any single ingredient.

Make It a Game: 5 points
Eat Your Colors: Green, Yellow / Orange

Invite Exploration

"What other ingredients could we add to our fruit crisp to try new flavors?"

Mini Pear-Apple Crisp

This recipe is forgiving and flexible. Add more or less fruit depending on your preference (or your child's interest in peeling and chopping)—it will be delicious no matter which way you make it. It's also easy to prepare ahead. Simply assemble the mini crisps in the individual ramekins, cover tightly, and store in the refrigerator for up to two days. When ready, just bake and enjoy!

PREP TIME: 20 minutes

COOK TIME: 30 to 35 minutes

Serves 12

INGREDIENTS:

FOR THE FILLING:

6 medium Anjou pears

4 medium Granny Smith apples

¾ cup dried cranberries

2 tablespoons fresh lemon juice (from 1 lemon)

¼ cup whole wheat all-purpose flour

½ cup honey

¼ teaspoon ground cinnamon

¼ teaspoon ground nutmeg

FOR THE TOPPING:

1¼ cups whole wheat all-purpose flour

1 cup old-fashioned rolled oats

16 tablespoons (2 sticks) unsalted butter, cold, cut into chunks

¼ cup flax meal

½ cup light brown sugar

DIRECTIONS:

1 Preheat the oven to 350°F.

2 To make the filling, peel and core the pears and apples, then cut them into large chunks. (I find this to be a tedious step, but my kids love recipes with lots of peeling and chopping so they were in charge. Don't worry about being too exact. Peel and chop as much fruit as your kids would like. The measurements don't need to be perfect, just in the ballpark.)

3 In a large bowl, combine the chopped fruit, cranberries, lemon juice, flour, honey, and spices. Using a large spoon, mix gently to combine. Set aside.

Cook Together

Beginners: Peel the fruit. Mix the crumble topping. Assemble the mini crisps.

Experts: Dice the fruit.

Tip: Do the peeling together (step 1), then divide up the remaining steps of this recipe to give each person a job. For example, with a family of four, each person can do one step. If the kids are taking the lead with Mom or Dad assisting, use the "Heads or Tails" method. Each child picks whether they are heads or tails. "Heads" are even numbers, "Tails" are odd. Toss a coin to see who goes first, divide up the steps, and start cooking!

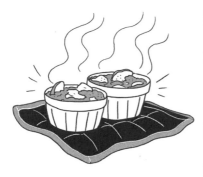

4 To make the topping, in a separate large bowl, combine the flour, oats, butter, flax meal, and sugar. Using your hands, mix the dough together until it looks like large crumbles. For younger kids, it's easier to divide the mixture into two smaller bowls. Work over a rimmed baking sheet to contain the mess.

5 Place 12 small ramekins on a rimmed baking sheet. Portion the fruit mixture evenly into the ramekins.

6 Top each ramekin with a handful of the crumble topping.

7 Bake for 30 to 35 minutes, or until the topping is lightly browned and the fruit is tender and bubbling.

8 Serve warm.

Buy in Season When pears are in season, your local farmers' market will boast a wide variety to choose from. Ask the farmer which pears are best for baking versus eating raw, and which variety she enjoys the most. Fill your basket with a selection of shapes and colors, and compare tastes and textures.

Pear and Parsnip Soup with Walnuts

This savory soup is another easy way to feature pears on your menu when they are in season. It's also a simple way to add some variety to your holiday table—a great alternative to Easy Butternut Squash Soup (page 95).

PREP TIME: 15 minutes

COOK TIME: 30 minutes

Serves 8

INGREDIENTS:

2 large Anjou pears (about
1 pound)

2 large Granny Smith apples
(about 1 pound)

2 large parsnips (about
1 pound)

1 medium white onion

¼ cup extra-virgin olive oil

1 teaspoon kosher salt

3 cups Chicken Broth
(page 99)

Chopped walnuts, for garnish

DIRECTIONS:

1 Preheat the oven to 450°F.

2 Peel the pears, apples, parsnips, and onion, then cut them into large wedges. Place on a rimmed baking sheet and toss with the oil and salt.

3 Bake, turning occasionally, for 20 to 25 minutes, or until golden brown.

4 Remove from the oven and let the mixture cool slightly. Working in batches, transfer the mixture to a blender with the broth and 1 cup water. Puree gently. It's best to work in small batches.

5 Transfer the soup to a medium stockpot and rewarm it over low heat.

6 Serve with a garnish of chopped walnuts.

Tip To get a more brothlike texture, add an extra ½ cup chicken broth when rewarming the soup.

Recipe inspired by my food friend and fellow mom Melissa Lanz of the Fresh 20.

Persimmons

The best analogy I can use for how our healthy eating habits look around the holidays is sledding. Huddled together on our wooden toboggan, we start off the season at a slow, gentle glide. As we hit the Halloween drop-off, our little sled gets a big push and we pick up some serious speed. Rolling into November, the hill gets steeper and our momentum continues right into Thanksgiving—my kids giddy with laughter, shouting, "Faster!" By December, we're careening down the steepest part of the hill at full tilt—sugar-covered cookies, candies, and cakes at every meal—and I feel like I've lost control. The kids are loving it, and I'm hanging on for dear life.

Our holiday table needed an overhaul. So I focused on finding a few healthy alternatives to round out our menu—dial back the frequency of the sugar bombs in our rotation, and feature a seasonal food that we hadn't yet tried. I started with persimmons.

A beautiful seasonal fruit, persimmons fit nicely with our family agreement to enjoy more fruits (in place of processed sugary treats) for dessert. They were a new food for my husband, my kids, and me, so we all had fun experimenting with how to enjoy them. They're also a great source of vitamins A and C, which was an added bonus. It turns out persimmons are a little low on the popularity scale, so the farmers at our market were overjoyed when we started buying them. When we baked them with cinnamon, ginger, and honey, the smell told us we had a winner before the first bite. Happiness filled our whole house, along with our bellies. They're equally delicious sliced like an apple or baked into chips.

Make It a Game: 5 points
Eat Your Colors: Yellow/Orange

Invite Exploration

"What do you notice about the pattern inside a persimmon?"

"I wonder what other fruits and vegetables have a beautiful pattern inside?"

"In what ways are apples like persimmons?"

Baked Persimmons

The deep orange hue of persimmons adds beautiful color to your fall table. Baked with cinnamon, ginger, and honey, this recipe makes a festive and healthy addition to your lineup of holiday treats—a nice alternative to baked apples.

PREP TIME: 5 minutes
COOK TIME: 40 to 50 minutes
Serves 8

INGREDIENTS:

4 medium Fuyu persimmons
2 tablespoons honey
½ teaspoon ground cinnamon
¼ teaspoon ground ginger

Cook Together

Beginners: Mix the dressing.

Experts: Cut the persimmons.

DIRECTIONS:

1 Preheat the oven to 350°F. Line a baking dish with foil.

2 Cut the tops off the persimmons. Cut the fruit in half horizontally through the middle, revealing the beautiful pattern inside. Place the cut fruit, flesh-side up, in the lined baking dish.

3 In a small saucepan, heat 1 cup water to a gentle boil. Add the honey, cinnamon, and ginger, reduce the heat, and simmer, mixing gently, for 2 minutes, or until the honey dissolves.

4 Pour the honey mixture over the persimmons, reserving some for serving. Cover and bake for 40 to 50 minutes, or until the fruit is soft.

5 Serve in small bowls with a drizzle of the honey-cinnamon syrup.

Buy in Season There is a big difference in flavor between the two main types of persimmons: the Fuyu and the Hachiya. Fuyus should be firm, and can be eaten whole like apples. Hachiyas need to be almost mushy before you can eat them—they are generally best for baking into cakes and cookies.

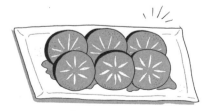

Persimmon Cake

Traditionally called persimmon pudding, this cake is an easy and delicious way to try Hachiya persimmons.

PREP TIME: 20 minutes

COOK TIME: 60 minutes

Serves 8

INGREDIENTS:

2 cups Hachiya persimmon pulp (from 6 to 8 persimmons)

4 large eggs, beaten

½ cup light brown sugar

16 tablespoons (2 sticks) unsalted butter, melted

2 teaspoons pure vanilla extract

2 cups whole wheat all-purpose flour

1 teaspoon baking soda

1 teaspoon ground cinnamon

½ teaspoon ground nutmeg

½ teaspoon kosher salt

Vanilla ice cream, for serving

DIRECTIONS:

1   Preheat the oven to 350°F. Lightly spray a large pie dish with olive oil.

2   In a large bowl combine the persimmon pulp, eggs, sugar, butter, and vanilla.

3   In a separate bowl, whisk together the flour, baking soda, cinnamon, nutmeg, and salt.

4   Working in small batches, add the dry ingredients to the wet ingredients and stir gently to combine. Pour the mixture into the prepared dish.

5   Bake for 60 minutes, or until the cake is firm but moist and a thin crust forms on top.

6   Serve warm with scoops of vanilla ice cream.

Tip   Add a handful of coarsely chopped walnuts for an extra boost of omega-3 oils and a delicious crunch!

Cook Together

Getting the pulp out of a Hachiya persimmon is a super project for kids of all ages and skill levels—but it's messy! The persimmons should be squishy when you hold them in your hand. Work over a rimmed baking sheet. Slice off the tops. Using a spoon, scoop out the insides of the persimmon and load the pulp into a large bowl. Encourage your kids to get their hands right into the mix to break up the large chunks.

Persimmon Chips

Follow the recipe for Apple Chips (page 104), substituting four Fuyu persimmons for the Granny Smith apples. Cooking time will vary slightly based on the water content in your persimmons as well as the thickness of the slices of fruit, so bake a little longer, if necessary. James absolutely loves the sweet and chewy flavor of these simple treats. They make a great lunchbox snack.

Keep Trying Even if your kids don't like the taste of persimmon, focus on the magical pattern that they reveal inside. Count the seeds inside a persimmon—the pattern reveals a Fibonacci number (see page 138). Read A Mathematical Menu section on page 138 for more clues to uncovering this magical pattern, then head out to the market to find it.

Pomegranates

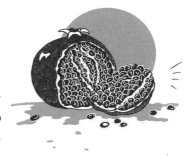

On my bad days, I find myself nagging Catherine to stop picking at her plate. On my good days, I accept that she likes to explore her food—first by touching, then by smelling, and finally working up to tasting. Instead of doing this at the dinner table, I set up ways for Catherine to explore new foods without the pressure of table manners, like at a sensing bar (see Explore Food with Your Five Senses on page 53).

Pomegranate is a perfect food for sensory exploration. Its rough exterior is an interesting tactile experience in and of itself, but hidden inside is a delicate treat—bright red juicy seeds that are perfect for picking with little fingers. Bonus: They're a great source of fiber, vitamin C, and vitamin K.[7] Although Catherine is happy to slice open a pomegranate and pick out the seeds, one by one, until her fingertips are as red as the fruit, our experience became even more fun when we discovered a clever, and mess-free way, of seeding a pomegranate.

All it took was a bowl of cold water. It was the perfect combination for us—Catherine could use her hands, and the control freak in me could relax knowing that my white countertops wouldn't turn pink from pomegranate juice stains. The experience of eating the seeds was great fun, too. The small red gems weren't daunting—just pick a little one to try—and the crunchy pops of tart flavor made a delicious after-school snack.

Make It a Game: 5 points
Eat Your Colors: Red

> ### Invite Exploration
>
> "I wonder why the seeds of a pomegranate sink, but the seeds of a pumpkin float?"
>
> "What other ways could we get the seeds out of a pomegranate?"

Poppin' Pomegranate Sauce

Pomegranate seeds are delicious simply on their own, but to try something new, we used them to remake an old favorite: cranberry sauce. Combined with cranberries and orange zest, pomegranate sauce was a welcome newcomer to our holiday table. It's also delicious paired with Easy Roasted Chicken (page 282) or Gigi's Roasted Pork Tenderloin (page 286) to dress up a weekday dinner.

PREP TIME: 5 minutes

COOK TIME: 10 to 15 minutes

Makes about 2 cups

INGREDIENTS:

½ cup honey

12 ounces fresh cranberries (about 4 cups)

1 tablespoon freshly squeezed orange juice

1 pomegranate, seeded (about 1 cup seeds; see page 115 for tips)

Orange zest, for garnish

DIRECTIONS:

1 In a small saucepan, combine the honey, cranberries, orange juice, and 1 cup water and bring to a gentle boil over medium heat. Reduce the heat and simmer for 15 minutes, or until the cranberries pop open and the mixture looks a little like jam.

2 Transfer to a small bowl, stir in the pomegranate seeds, and garnish with orange zest.

Cook Together

Beginners: Break apart the pomegranate and separate the seeds in a big bowl of water.

Experts: Cut the pomegranate.

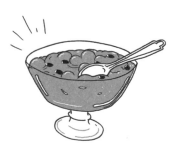

Wild Rice with Pomegranate and Pistachios

Mixing pomegranate seeds with rice is another easy way to feature this fruit on your family table. If your kids resist the nutty flavor of wild rice in this dish, use the Work-Your-Way-Up Strategy (see page 56).

PREP TIME: 10 minutes

COOK TIME: 20 minutes

Serves 4

INGREDIENTS:

1 cup wild rice (or substitute brown rice)

2 cups water or Chicken Broth (page 99)

½ cup pomegranate seeds (see below for tips)

¼ cup coarsely chopped pistachios

Handful of fresh parsley leaves

Kosher salt

DIRECTIONS:

1 In a medium saucepan, combine the wild rice with the water or broth. Bring to a boil over medium-high heat, then reduce the heat to low and simmer for 20 minutes, or until the liquid has been absorbed. The rice can also be made in a rice cooker.

2 In a large bowl, combine the cooked rice, pomegranate seeds, pistachios, and parsley. Season with kosher salt to taste.

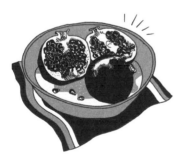

The No-Mess Way to Seed a Pomegranate

Pomegranate seeds are delicious, but they can be messy. The no-mess trick is to immerse the fruit in a big bowl of cold water, then break apart the membranes with your fingers. Lots of seeds, less mess.

1. Slice the pomegranate in half and place it in a large bowl of cold water.
2. Working under the water, break apart the fruit using your fingers to release the pomegranate seeds from the membrane.
3. Like magic, the membranes float to the top and the seeds sink to the bottom.
4. Pour off the membrane-filled water, rinse the seeds in a sieve, and you've got a beautiful batch of seeds ready to snack on. You can also use them in salads and sauces.

Whole Wheat Flour

For my family, the easiest way to get started cooking together was baking. Scooping, mixing, and pouring represent the trifecta of easy family cooking. And the sweet surprise at the end provided a delicious reward. Although a big part of the 52 New Foods Challenge is learning to cook a wide variety of dishes together and move beyond baking, I would be lying if I pretended that my kids' favorite cooking projects didn't involve sweet treats. But baking introduces a villain to our story: refined flour.

According to the USDA, we're allocating more than three times the recommended amount of our food budgets to refined grains and less than 20 percent of the ideal source: whole grains.[8] This is a problem because refined grains leave out the good stuff (nutrient-rich bran and germ) in favor of the not-so-good stuff (mostly starch).[9]

So just use whole-grain flour, right?

For most kids, including mine, it takes time to adjust to the flavor and texture of whole wheat flour. That's when you use the Work-Your-Way-Up Strategy (see page 56). Instead of forcing the issue, slowly work whole wheat flour into your recipes—increasing the amount in small increments each time you make the dish. A great way to start experimenting is with simple recipes like crepes, pancakes, and pizza.

Make It a Game: 5 points
Eat Your Colors: Healthy Grains

Invite Exploration

"What other recipes could we remake using whole wheat flour?"

Healthy Crepes

Crepes are an easy and fun way to cook with your kids! My kids love them hot off the pan, but they can easily be made ahead to save time on busy mornings. This recipe also makes it easy to shift to whole-grain flour. With Strawberry Sauce (page 209) or Warm Cinnamon Apples (page 103) tucked inside and a touch of real maple syrup, you'll never miss the refined flour.

PREP TIME: 5 minutes

COOK TIME: 15 minutes

Serves 4

INGREDIENTS:

1 cup whole wheat all-purpose flour

¼ teaspoon kosher salt

1¾ cups nonfat milk

3 large eggs, beaten

3 tablespoons unsalted butter, melted and slightly cooled

Fresh fruit, Greek yogurt, honey, or Strawberry Sauce (page 209), for serving

Cook Together

Beginners: Scoop. Mix. Pour.

Experts: Swirl the batter in the pan.

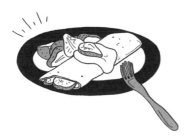

DIRECTIONS:

1   In a large bowl, whisk together the flour and salt.

2   In a separate large bowl, whisk together the milk, eggs, and melted butter.

3   Working in small batches, add the flour mixture to the egg mixture, stirring gently.

4   Warm a small frying pan over medium heat. Lightly spray with olive oil. Add ¼ cup of the batter, swirling quickly to evenly coat the pan with a thin layer of batter. Work with two pans to speed things up and avoid fights over who gets to swirl the batter!

5   Cook for 2 to 3 minutes, or until the underside of the crepe is golden brown. Flip the crepe and cook for 2 minutes more.

6   Serve warm, with fresh fruit, a dollop of Greek yogurt, and a drizzle of honey, real maple syrup, or Strawberry Sauce (page 209).

Tip *Swirling is the most important part of this recipe. If the batter sets before spreading in the pan, the crepes will be too thick. It's also a great job for more experienced kids—swirling is so much fun! Holding the handle of the pan with two hands, slowly rotate your wrist in a clockwise, circular motion, gently swirling the batter to the outside edges of the pan.*

Instead of fruit and yogurt, add a fried egg, slice of ham, and a sprinkle of mozzarella and turn these breakfast crepes into dinner. Pair with Crispy Sweet Potato Fries (page 66) and Brussels Sprouts Chips (page 77) to round out your colors.

Banana Pancakes

Making pancakes with Daddy is a favorite cooking activity for my kids. Plus, it's another easy recipe to work your way up (see page 56). If your kids aren't used to the flavor and texture of whole wheat flour, adjust the amount you use in small increments each time you make this recipe.

PREP TIME: 10 minutes

COOK TIME: 15 minutes

Serves 4

INGREDIENTS:

1 cup whole wheat all-purpose flour

1 teaspoon baking powder

½ teaspoon baking soda

¼ teaspoon kosher salt

1 cup nonfat milk

1 large egg, beaten

1 tablespoon unsalted butter, melted and slightly cooled

1 large banana

DIRECTIONS:

1 Preheat a griddle to 350°F.

2 In a small bowl, mix together the flour, baking powder, baking soda, and salt.

3 In a separate bowl, beat together the milk, egg, and melted butter. In small batches, add the flour mixture to the egg mixture. Stir gently until combined.

4 Spray the griddle with olive oil. Using a small measuring cup, pour the batter onto the heated griddle. Each pancake should be about the size of your child's palm. Add a few slices of banana on top of each pancake.

5 Cook for 2 to 3 minutes. When bubbles begin to appear on the pancake's surface, flip and cook for 2 to 3 minutes more, or until golden brown on the second side.

Whole Wheat Pizza Dough

It's easier to buy pizza dough premade, but making it yourself is a super-fun activity for your kids—like play clay. Save this project for a weekend, when you can relax and enjoy the time cooking with your kids.

PREP TIME: 15 minutes

WAIT TIME: 5 hours

Makes 2 crusts

INGREDIENTS:

1¾ cups warm water

1 tablespoon extra-virgin olive oil

2 teaspoons kosher salt

1½ teaspoons active dry yeast

4¼ cups whole wheat all-purpose flour

DIRECTIONS:

1 In a large bowl, whisk together the warm water, oil, salt, and yeast.

2 Place the bowl on a rimmed baking sheet. Add the flour and mix the dough with a wooden spoon. Once the dough is mostly combined, knead the dough like play clay. (For some kids, it's easiest to take the dough out of the bowl and work on the baking sheet.) Keep mixing until the dough is thoroughly combined and comes together into a ball without sticking to your hands. Add a little extra flour if the dough is sticky.

3 Cover the bowl, leaving a small section uncovered to allow the gases to escape. Set the bowl on the counter for 2 hours to let the dough rise.

4 Refrigerate the risen dough for at least 3 hours before using.

5 Divide the dough into 2 large balls. Each ball makes one crust. If not using immediately, wrap in plastic wrap and keep in the refrigerator for up to 1 week or in the freezer for up to 1 month.

> **Keep Trying** My kids were slow to warm to the flavor and texture of whole wheat flour. Work your way up in small steps—and keep trying!

Winter

Kale

Kale is making a comeback. This leafy green vegetable is quickly gaining ground on the nutrition popularity charts. And for good reason. The health benefits of kale are solid: It's a great source of vitamins K, C, and A, and its deep green color is an indication of the antioxidants it packs. All good. But there are even bigger benefits that kale offers, beyond the nutrition facts.

First, it's a great way to transition your kids away from unhealthy snacks. Instead of taking potato chips away, I invited a healthy alternative to our table: kale chips. With a salty flavor reminiscent of potato chips and a crunchy, crumbly texture like dried seaweed, kale chips were an instant success. Like potato chips, you can never eat just one. Once comfortably seated in a top-ten favorite foods slot, it wasn't hard to wean us from potato chips—we still crave them some days, but that craving is easily staved off with a big bowl of crunchy, colorful kale chips.

Second, it's a great vegetable to cook with your kids. Catherine and James love tearing the big, bold leaves of kale to make recipes that feature this nutritional rock star. No special (or dangerous) kitchen tools required. Experimenting with seasonings for our Crispy Kale Chips—cumin, paprika, and garlic powder being the current favorites—is another easy way to let my kids lead in the kitchen.

So when you consider kale and its benefits, look beyond nutrition. The cooking adventures it inspires are the real benefit to the health of your family.

Make It a Game: 15 points
Eat Your Colors: Green, Red

Invite Exploration

"How does the flavor of kale change when it's raw versus when it's roasted?"

Crispy Kale Chips

Packed with nutrients, a big batch of kale chips is a colorful, healthy snack that's easy to make. Bonus: They beat back cravings for unhealthy snacks. These chips are easy enough for a five-year-old to prepare and a dish that the whole family can enjoy, which wins them (even) more points in my book. Bet you can't eat just one!

PREP TIME: 10 minutes

COOK TIME: 25 to 30 minutes

Serves 4

INGREDIENTS:

1 bunch curly kale

1 tablespoon extra-virgin olive oil

¼ teaspoon kosher salt

Cook Together

Beginners: Tear the leaves from the stalks. Wash the leaves. Massage the leaves.

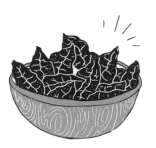

DIRECTIONS:

1   Remove the stems and tough center ribs from each leaf of kale. Tear the large leaves into smaller pieces. Wash the leaves, spin them in a salad spinner to remove the water, and set aside on paper towels to dry thoroughly— this is the key to making super-crunchy kale chips. It's even better if you can do this step a day ahead to let the leaves dry fully.

2   Preheat the oven to 250°F.

3   Place the kale on a rimmed baking sheet. Add the oil and salt and massage them into the leaves. The color of the leaves will change from dusty to deep green, which is how you'll know they are adequately coated. Arrange the leaves in a single, even layer on the pan. If you have a particularly large bunch of kale, use two pans.

4   Bake for 25 to 30 minutes, or until crispy.

5   Serve immediately.

Tip *Cooking time will vary based on how much moisture is in the leaves. Watch carefully at about 20 minutes to be sure your chips don't burn.*

Keep Trying Try Crispy Kale Chips with a few different seasonings. Garlic powder, cumin, and paprika are great options. You can also try them with different varieties of kale, then compare tastes and textures.

Sautéed Kale and Cranberries

This is a colorful side dish that I like to serve with Easy Roasted Chicken (page 282) or Anthony's Famous Short Ribs (page 285). It's also a great way to try a different texture (and flavor) of kale. Let your kids tear the leaves for this recipe—it's an easy way to get them involved in making dinner together.

PREP TIME: 10 minutes

COOK TIME: 5 minutes

Serves 4

INGREDIENTS:

1 large bunch curly kale

1 tablespoon extra-virgin olive oil

1 clove garlic, finely chopped

¼ cup dried cranberries or dried currants

¼ teaspoon kosher salt

Grow It Kale is hardy and easy to grow. It will tolerate colder temperatures. Plant in late summer for a fall or early winter harvest.

DIRECTIONS:

1 Prepare the kale. Remove the stems and tough center ribs from each leaf of kale. Tear the large leaves into smaller pieces. Wash and dry the leaves.

2 Heat a large sauté pan over medium heat. Add the oil and garlic and sauté for 30 seconds. Add the kale and sauté for 3 minutes more, or until the leaves turn deep green and wilt. Add a little water if the pan seems dry.

3 Add the cranberries and salt. Toss in the pan to combine.

4 Serve warm.

Make It a Main

Before sautéing the kale, add 2 cups chickpeas to the oil and garlic in the pan. Cook for 5 minutes, or until the chickpeas begin to brown. Add the kale and ½ cup water or Chicken Broth (page 99) to the pan and cook 5 minutes more. Finish with the cranberries and salt. Serve over brown rice.

Buy in Season Look for lots of different varieties at your local farmers' market including red kale, curly kale, and lacinato (dinosaur) kale. If you sign up for a weekly CSA (community supported agriculture) delivery, kale will dominate your box between January and March.

Radicchio

Radicchio may be loaded with antioxidants—its deep, purplish-red color being the telltale sign—but it's equally loaded with bitterness. It reminds me of those beautiful holiday dresses with the billowing tulle skirts. I love the way they look, but getting Catherine to actually wear one for more than five minutes is another story. This fancy lettuce may be a beautiful complement to salads and savory pasta dishes, but it can be incredibly challenging to get kids to try.

That is, unless you roast it.

Catherine's preference for crispiness was what led us down this path. All of the recipes we tried where radicchio was the main event were rather bitter and unappealing. What would happen if we sliced the radicchio extra thin, into long, ruffle-edged strips, and roasted it? Like garlic, kale, and cauliflower, the flavor of radicchio mellows after a quick roast in the oven. It loses some of its beautiful color, but in return it delivers a rich, nutty flavor that my kids can't resist. Catherine named them Ridiculous Radicchio Chips.

Another easy way to work this new food into your meals is with a DIY dinner. Instead of radicchio being the main feature on your menu, pair it with a series of other favorite foods and invite your kids to make their own mix. Encourage them to add just a sprinkle—a taster—of thinly shaved radicchio. Ask everyone to make one dish for themselves, and two to share. Then trade. Force your kids to try radicchio and they will resist. Let them lead and you'll find that they will be open to experimenting.

Make It a Game: 15 points
Eat Your Colors: Blue/Purple

Invite Exploration

"How would you make a salad to maximize your points?"

"Can you make a salad using all of the colors on the table?"

DIY Rainbow Salad

The power of the DIY Rainbow Salad bar is the comfort in knowing you can try new foods on your own terms. It's a great way to introduce challenging new foods, like radicchio. Encourage your kids to try even a few small sprinkles of radicchio or a couple of jícama matchsticks. It's 100 percent okay if they don't like it on the first try. Keep trying!

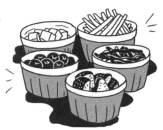

PREP TIME: 20 minutes

COOK TIME: 0 minutes

Serves 4

INGREDIENTS:

3 rainbow carrots

2 tomatillos

1 jícama

1 avocado

1 mango

1 pint strawberries

½ pint blueberries

½ head radicchio

5 slices pineapple

1 small onion

1 Meyer lemon or lime

Fresh cilantro, for garnish

Tip If you choose to include tomatillos in your salad bar, consider roasting them first. Ten minutes in a 350°F oven will do the trick. My kids were more open to the flavor of roasted tomatillo than the raw version, although you can serve it either way.

DIRECTIONS:

1 Peel and dice your veggies and fruits.

2 Place each of your ingredients in a small bowl and line them up in the colors of the rainbow. You should have between ½ cup and 1 cup of each ingredient.

3 Let each person create their own recipe. Encourage everyone to include at least three colors in their mix. Bonus points for trying any of the new foods, even just a taster.

4 To finish, squeeze a little Meyer lemon or lime on top of your salad and garnish with cilantro.

Cook Together

Beginners: Arrange ingredients into bowls by color. Assemble salads to share.

Experts: Chop the vegetables.

Tip: Let your kids do as much of the prep as possible. My only exception is with using the mandoline, a utensil with a sharp blade for making very thin slices of ingredients. To create super-thin shreds of radicchio, as well as jícama and carrot matchsticks, I prefer to use a mandoline. I'm not brave enough to let my kids have at it with that slicer—at least not until I find a safer version! Everything else is fair game.

Ridiculous Radicchio Chips

This recipe is a great example of how a food fail turned into a family favorite. Experimenting with roasted radicchio wedges, we decided it would be easier to shred the leaves. The result was these delicious, nutty chips that remind me of the crispy onions used to garnish mashed potatoes. My kids love them!

PREP TIME: 10 minutes

COOK TIME: 25 minutes

Serves 4

INGREDIENTS:

1 head radicchio

1 tablespoon extra-virgin olive oil

½ teaspoon kosher salt

DIRECTIONS:

1 Preheat the oven to 400°F.

2 Slice the radicchio into ¼-inch sections. Pull apart the leaves and cut any large pieces into small strips.

3 Toss on a rimmed baking sheet with the oil and salt. Arrange the slices in a single, even layer on the pan.

4 Roast for 25 minutes, turning once, until the strips are brown and crispy.

Invite Exploration Catherine's preference for almost-burnt chips, like Crispy Kale Chips (page 124) and Brussels Sprouts Chips (page 77), led us to Ridiculous Radicchio Chips. We sliced the radicchio extra thin and roasted it until crispy, and it was a hit! My kids ate it straight from the pan—then asked for seconds. I never would have known had I not followed Catherine's lead and experimented with textures based on her preferences.

Buy in Season See if you can spot two different kinds of radicchio at your local market. One will be shaped like a cabbage, with a round head. The other looks more like romaine lettuce, with long, slender leaves.

Keep Trying Radicchio tends to be bitter, which can be problematic for picky palates. Roasting calms the bitterness, which makes it easier for finicky eaters to give it a try. Don't worry if your kids don't like it right away—this food takes some time to grow on you (adults included). Enjoying the pleasures of cooking together is more important than whether they eat what you make.

Bok Choy

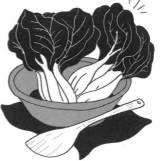

If phase one of our eating adventure was defined by the three Ps—pasta, pizza, and peas—phase two was dominated by the big B: broccoli. Broccoli soon became a vegetable I could rely on. With the occasional nudge, my kids would eat it without much fuss. Make no mistake, I was happy that we were eating healthier.

But at a certain point, a landscape dominated by "mini trees" gets boring, no matter what you call them. Even more, you can't rely on a narrow stable of fruits and vegetables if you're trying to eat healthy. The key is variety.

How did we get beyond broccoli? Bok choy!

Step one was to start small. The target: a mild-flavored but colorful vegetable, with a somewhat leafy texture, but not so bold as to scare away small children. Mild mannered, both in color and taste, bok choy met all of my starter requirements and, to its further benefit, could easily be mixed into our favorite stir-fries and soups. Once my kids warmed up to bok choy in some of their favorite dishes, we moved to trying it solo.

Using favorite foods as a vehicle for trying something new is a key strategy that will help your kids branch out (see page 57). Start with working bok choy into something simple and tasty like a savory rice and chicken dish: our Clay-Pot Chicken with Bok Choy (page 130) is a fan favorite. Slowly work your way up to trying bok choy without the vehicle. Letting your kids add "sprinkles" (aka sesame seeds) to your sautéed bok choy is another way to make it fun.

Make It a Game: 15 points
Eat Your Colors: Green

> ### Invite Exploration
> "What other vegetables does bok choy remind you of? What gives you that idea?"

Clay-Pot Chicken with Bok Choy

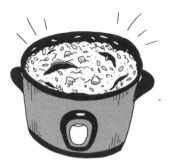

This simple recipe is an easy version of one of my favorite Asian comfort foods: clay-pot chicken. Though not made in a traditional clay pot, this recipe delivers a big, cozy umami flavor with very little effort. One of my go-to weeknight recipes, it's easy to prepare, tastes delicious, and can make an encore appearance in your lunchbox the next day.

PREP TIME: 10 minutes

WAIT TIME: 60 minutes (optional)

COOK TIME: 30 to 40 minutes

Serves 4

INGREDIENTS:

4 bunches baby bok choy

2 cloves garlic, minced

1 tablespoon mirin (optional)

¼ cup tamari or soy sauce

¼ teaspoon Chinese five-spice

1 tablespoon honey

1 pound boneless chicken thighs, trimmed and diced into ½-inch pieces

2 cups long-grain brown rice

1 tablespoon grapeseed oil

DIRECTIONS:

1   Chop the bok choy into 1- to 2-inch sections. Separate the stalks from the leaves (the stalks go into the pot first because they take longer to cook). Discard the ends.

2   In a medium bowl, whisk together the garlic, mirin, tamari, five-spice, and honey. Add the chicken and stir to coat evenly.

3   In the bowl of a rice cooker, rinse the rice, then add enough water to cover the rice by 1 inch and set to cook (about 15 minutes). If using a saucepan, bring 4 cups water and the rice to a boil, then reduce the heat to medium and simmer for 20 minutes or until almost all of the liquid has been absorbed and the rice is fluffy. (My preference is for the rice cooker as it's infinitely more reliable.)

Cook Together

Beginners: Give the bok choy a bath.

Experts: Chop the leaves into large sections.

Tip: Bok choy can be dirty. After chopping the leaves, soak them in a large bowl filled with water. Have your kids swish the leaves gently in the water, then let the leaves stand for a few minutes. The dirt will sink to the bottom, while the leaves float to the top.

Keep Trying

If your kids don't like brown rice, use the Work-Your-Way-Up Strategy (see page 56).

4   While the rice is cooking, heat a wok or large sauté pan over medium-high heat. Add the oil, then the marinated chicken and sauté, stirring occasionally, for about 7 minutes, or until the chicken is crispy on the edges and bounces back gently when pressed with a fork.

5   Just before the rice is finished, add the stalks of the bok choy leaves to the rice cooker or pot, depending on which you are using. Cover and let cook for 3 minutes. Add the remaining bok choy leaves and the chicken, cover, and cook for 2 minutes more, or until the leaves are slightly wilted and bright green.

6   Gently mix the bok choy, chicken, and rice together to combine. The bok choy will continue to wilt as you stir.

7   Serve warm in a large bowl, family style.

Tip *For better flavor, cover and marinate the chicken for 1 hour before cooking.*

Sizzling Bok Choy

This is a quick-and-easy side dish that I like to pair with Pan-Seared Tofu Slices (page 288) or Ginger-Soy Glazed Cod (page 287). Let your kids add "sprinkles"—aka sesame seeds—before serving.

PREP TIME: 5 minutes

COOK TIME: 5 minutes

Serves 4

INGREDIENTS:

4 bunches baby bok choy

2 tablespoons grapeseed oil

½ teaspoon finely chopped peeled fresh ginger

½ teaspoon finely chopped garlic

1 teaspoon tamari or soy sauce

Sesame seeds, for garnish

DIRECTIONS:

1 Chop the bok choy into 1-inch sections. Discard the ends.

2 Heat a large wok or sauté pan over medium heat. Add the oil, ginger, and garlic and sauté for 30 seconds, or until the garlic and ginger are just fragrant.

3 Add the bok choy and cook for 3 to 5 minutes, or until the leaves are bright green with slightly brown edges.

4 Add the tamari or soy sauce and toss gently in the pan to coat.

5 Garnish with sesame seeds before serving.

Cinnamon Beef Noodle Soup with Bok Choy

This is my favorite winter dish. The smell of cinnamon and beef simmering is cozy and comforting. It's also a great way to try a variety of leafy green vegetables—bok choy, spinach, and kale all work well with this recipe.

PREP TIME: 15 minutes

COOK TIME: 90 minutes

Serves 4

INGREDIENTS:

1 tablespoon grapeseed oil

4 cloves garlic, smashed

4 coins fresh ginger

½ cup tamari or soy sauce

2 pounds beef stew meat, cut into 1-inch cubes

2 cinnamon sticks

2 star anise pods

½ pound noodles, such as udon or fettuccine

4 cups bok choy leaves, ends discarded

Scallions, for garnish

DIRECTIONS:

1 Heat a large stockpot over medium-high heat. Add the oil, garlic, and ginger. Sauté for 30 seconds, or until the mixture is fragrant.

2 Add the tamari, beef, cinnamon sticks, star anise, and 8 cups water. Bring the mixture to a boil, then reduce the heat to low, cover, and simmer for 90 minutes, or until the beef is tender. The longer you cook the meat, the softer it will become.

3 While the soup is cooking, bring a large pot of water to a boil and prepare the noodles according to the package directions. Cook until just tender, drain, then set aside.

4 Remove the ginger, garlic, star anise, and cinnamon sticks from the soup. Skim the surface to remove any fat. Add the bok choy leaves. Bring the soup back to a boil and cook for 2 minutes more, or until the leaves are wilted.

5 Portion a small amount of cooked noodles into individual bowls, then ladle the soup over the noodles. Garnish with a sprinkle of chopped scallions.

Tip *This recipe can be made in a slow cooker set to low for 6 hours.*

Keep Trying If your kids resist big, leafy pieces of bok choy, try chopping them into smaller pieces and work your way up. Invite them to try the white parts of the bok choy versus the green parts to explore tastes and textures.

Romanesco

"Who can find something new to try?" That simple call to action changed our weekly shopping trip from a dreaded chore into a game for Catherine and James. Instead of hanging off the shopping cart, whining about how they would rather be playing, my kids happily took the lead scouting out new foods to try.

It didn't take long to spot an unusual newcomer, seemingly transported from a craggy planet in an alternate universe. If its vibrant chartreuse color hadn't caught their eyes, its mystical spiraling pattern certainly would have commanded their attention.

"Alien broccoli!" James exclaimed—arguably, a more cogent description of this fantastical food than its common name, Romanesco. Looking like a cross between broccoli and cauliflower, this fractal-pattern food arrives for a short spell each winter. We learned that it's actually a cousin of cauliflower, not broccoli, and has a similar flavor and texture and many of the same characteristics when you cook it. Don't miss it when it lands at your market—blink and, like a UFO, it will disappear.

As I talked about in Eat Your Colors (page 21), inviting your kids to go on a scavenger hunt at the market has myriad benefits. First, it puts them in charge of finding your new food of the week, shifting the ownership of your 52 New Foods Challenge from you to them. Second, it makes it easy for your kids to tune in to the terrific variety that each season brings. Instead of the same old (often boring) favorites, nature will deliver something refreshingly new, just when you need it. And everything is more interesting when it's available "for a limited time only!"

Make It a Game: 15 points
Eat Your Colors: Green

> ### Invite Exploration
>
> "Do you notice a pattern in this food? Which other foods have a similar pattern?"
>
> "Why do you think Romanesco grows this way?"

Roasted Romanesco

A spiraling spectacle, Romanesco resembles a cross between broccoli and cauliflower. Like its cousin cauliflower, it is delicious roasted with a touch of olive oil and salt. Bonus: It presents a fun math challenge. Can you find the pattern in its florets?

PREP TIME: 5 minutes

COOK TIME: 10 to 15 minutes

Serves 4

INGREDIENTS:

1 head Romanesco broccoli (sometimes called broccoflower)

2 tablespoons extra-virgin olive oil

½ teaspoon kosher salt

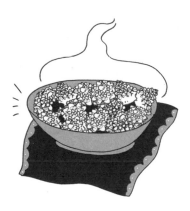

DIRECTIONS:

1 Preheat the oven to 375°F.

2 Wash and trim the Romanesco into small florets.

3 Place the florets on a rimmed baking sheet, add the oil and salt, and toss in the pan to coat evenly.

4 Bake, turning halfway through, for 10 to 15 minutes, or until the florets are browned.

Cook Together

Beginners: Using your hands, break apart the bunches of Romanesco into smaller florets.

Experts: Chop the florets.

Tip: To easily cut Romanesco, flip the head upside down and, using a paring knife, cut around the core to remove the stem. Break apart the large bunches and trim the small florets from the inner stems. Cut the florets in half again to make bite-size pieces.

Sautéed Romanesco with Lemon and Parmesan

Like cauliflower and Brussels sprouts, sautéing Romanesco is another way to experiment with its taste and texture. Use this recipe to let your kids compare the taste of Romanesco roasted versus sautéed. Note the differences and their preference.

PREP TIME: 10 minutes

COOK TIME: 10 minutes

Serves 4

INGREDIENTS:

1 tablespoon extra-virgin olive oil

2 cups chopped Romanesco (about ½-inch pieces)

¼ teaspoon kosher salt

1 tablespoon fresh lemon juice (from ½ lemon)

Grated Parmesan cheese, for garnish

DIRECTIONS:

1 Heat a large sauté pan over medium heat. Add the oil and Romanesco and cook, stirring occasionally, for 10 minutes, or until the Romanesco turns crispy on the edges. Add a little water to the pan if it looks dry while cooking.

2 Add the salt, lemon juice, and a dash of Parmesan cheese. Toss to combine.

3 Serve immediately.

Buy in Season Romanesco is available for only a few weeks each year, in the fall. Be on the lookout at your local market! Like cauliflower, look for firm, heavy heads.

A Mathematical Menu

My son, James, loves math. From a very early age he has been fascinated with numbers and has a special affinity for patterns of any kind. Like Catherine and her writing, I'm always trying to find ways to have James explore and experience food from different perspectives—ideally through the lens of his passion.

You can imagine James' delight when he discovered that there is a mathematical pattern in some foods: the Fibonacci sequence. This special sequence of numbers, discovered by Italian mathematician Leonardo Fibonacci, follows a predictable pattern: 0, 1, 1, 2, 3, 5, 8, 13, 21, 34, and so on. The numbers build on themselves—add the two proceeding numbers to determine the next. For example, $1 + 1 = 2$, then $1 + 2 = 3$, then $2 + 3 = 5$. What's fascinating is this pattern is evident in nature, including in many plant-based foods.

The spirals on a pineapple follow the Fibonacci sequence. Turn the pineapple upside down. Place your finger on the base of the first spiral and follow it diagonally out from the base. Continue counting the spirals around the bottom of the pineapple until you return to the place where you started. You'll always find a Fibonacci sequence. Slice open a persimmon and count the seeds. A Fibonacci sequence will be revealed. Magic! Once you start looking for it, you'll see it everywhere.

It would seem only appropriate, then, that Italian broccoli would display this pattern—an ode to the Italian mathematician who discovered the roots of this pattern. The Fibonacci sequence is more challenging to count on the tiny florets of a head of Romanesco, but its unmistakable fractal pattern is impossible to miss at the market.

As part of your 52 New Foods Challenge, look for math on your menu—whether it's a search for the Fibonacci sequence or simply counting fractions as you measure. It's another fun way to experience food from a new perspective, whether you've got a budding mathematician in your family or not.

Fibonacci Foods

Many foods reveal the magical Fibonnaci sequence. Check out these foods to see if you can find the pattern. Start by counting the seeds inside fruit, like apples. Then count the spirals on a pineapple or artichoke. Discover more and add to the list.

Apples
Artichokes
Brussels sprouts
Cauliflower
Grapefruits
Persimmons
Romanesco
Pineapples

Some other easy places to spot the Fibonacci sequence in nature:

Pinecones
Sunflowers

A special note of thanks to Peter Koehler, my son James's math teacher. Peter taught James about the Fibonacci sequence, and more important, set him on an adventure to find it in the world around him—including on his plate.

Edamame

Packing lunches that my kids will actually eat remains an elusive mystery. More often than not, Catherine will bring home lunches completely untouched. Her scuffling gait and glassy gaze in the late-afternoon pickup line at school are dead give-aways that she hasn't eaten lunch. I can tell even before she enters the car. Catherine's excuses are well crafted and endless. Not enough time. Too soggy. Too cold. Too mushy. Too hard to eat. Traded with a friend.

To give our lunches a boost, I sought help from my most reliable partner: edamame. Packed with protein, and a super source of folate, edamame beans are essential in our lunchboxes because: a) I know my kids will eat them, and b) they have enough power to help little bodies make it through the day. There are three simple variants I use for lunch, all featuring edamame: stir-fried rice, noodle soups, and pasta. These basic dishes can be prepared in myriad ways, and in each scenario, I load them with color—always aiming for three—to pack as much nutrition as I can into one thermos.

Edamame can be enjoyed straight from the pod—portability being one of its most endearing features. It can also be easily mixed into any one of our foundation dishes—it tastes equally great in a veggie stir-fry as it does in a soup or pasta dish. Frankly, the combination of color and protein in any bean makes it a great, all-purpose ingredient—but for my kids, the ease of edamame can't be beat. For a delicious snack, try it roasted. It's a salty, savory treat that is a great way to power back up after a long school day.

Make It a Game: 10 points
Eat Your Colors: Green and Protein

> ### Invite Exploration
> "What other ways could we work protein into your lunch?"

Power Lunch Veggie Stir-Fry

This easy stir-fry can be made with any leftover veggies you have in your fridge. It's one of our favorite lunchbox foundation dishes. Swap black beans for the edamame, tomato sauce for the tamari, add cilantro, and you've got a Southwestern-inspired dish.

PREP TIME: 10 minutes

COOK TIME: 5 minutes

Serves 4

INGREDIENTS:

1 tablespoon grapeseed oil

3 cups cooked long-grain brown rice

1 large egg, beaten

1 cup shelled edamame beans

½ cup finely chopped carrots

½ cup yellow corn kernels

2 tablespoons tamari or soy sauce

1 teaspoon sesame seeds

DIRECTIONS:

1 Heat a large wok or sauté pan over medium heat. Add the oil and rice and cook for 2 minutes, stirring frequently, or until the rice is slightly brown and crispy on the edges.

2 Create a well in the middle of the pan. Add the egg and cook, stirring occasionally with a heatproof spatula, for 2 minutes, or until the egg is almost cooked through.

3 Add the edamame, carrots, corn, and tamari to the rice mixture and combine. Cook for 1 minute more, or until the veggies begin to soften.

4 Garnish with sesame seeds and serve immediately, or pack in a thermos.

Cook Together

Beginners: Remove the beans from the pods. Crack the egg.

Experts: Sauté the ingredients in the wok.

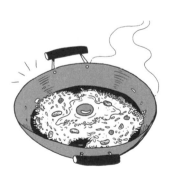

Roasted Edamame Pop'ems

This is one of our favorite healthy snacks. They are best served warm, right out of the oven.

PREP TIME: 5 minutes

COOK TIME: 40 minutes

Serves 4

INGREDIENTS:

1 pound frozen shelled edamame

1 tablespoon extra-virgin olive oil

½ teaspoon kosher salt

DIRECTIONS:

1 Preheat the oven to 375°F.

2 Place the frozen edamame in a strainer and run under warm water for a few minutes to remove ice clumps.

3 Transfer the edamame to a rimmed baking sheet. Pat dry with a paper towel to remove any excess water. Add the oil and salt to the beans, then toss to combine. Spread the beans into a single, even layer on the pan.

4 Roast, stirring occasionally, for 30 to 40 minutes, or until the beans turn golden brown and puffy.

5 Serve immediately. The beans will lose their crunchy texture as they cool.

Edamame Pasta Salad

Another lunchbox companion, this pasta dish is an easy way to work in your colors: green, yellow, and red.

PREP TIME: 5 minutes

COOK TIME: 10 minutes

Serves 4

INGREDIENTS:

1 pound fusilli pasta

1 cup frozen shelled edamame

½ cup cooked corn kernels

½ cup halved cherry tomatoes

2 tablespoons extra-virgin olive oil

1 tablespoon grated Parmesan cheese

Kosher salt

DIRECTIONS:

1 Bring a large pot of salted water to a boil, then cook the pasta according to the package directions. One minute before the pasta finishes cooking, add the frozen edamame. Drain and return to the pot.

2 Add the corn, tomatoes, oil, and cheese to the pasta and edamame. Stir to combine. Season with salt to taste.

3 Serve warm or cold.

Keep Trying Experiment with dishes served hot versus cold. To keep food warm, fill a thermos with hot water and let it stand for a few minutes. Pour out the water, then add the food. To keep food cold, add a small ice pack to the lunchbox before packing.

How to Build a Better Lunchbox

If you're like me, packing a healthy lunch that your kids will actually eat is one of the most challenging tasks you face each week. I was fed up (and fresh out of ideas). So, together with my kids, we came up with a simple strategy to build a better lunchbox. For a system of any kind to be successful in our house it has to be: a) sustainable (one that I can maintain on a busy schedule), and b) easy (one that my kids can be a part of). With those guiding principles, we came up with a few simple lunch-packing agreements.

1. Eat Your Colors
   The kids decided that the same principles we use to build balanced, healthy dinners could be used to build a healthy lunchbox: 3 colors + 1 protein + 1 healthy grain + 1 liquid. It's easy to remember and, with a little bit of practice, easy to achieve when building your box. Juicy red strawberries, sweet peas in nature's perfect package, and cheery pops of yellow cherry tomatoes. Red. Green. Yellow. Play with colors to make your box fun. No special shapes required.

2. Think Out of the Box
   School lunches can be the worst offenders when it comes to processed and overpackaged foods. Inspired by a project in my son's kindergarten class where the kids investigated the impact of trash on our oceans, James decided to make our lunch boxes 100 percent plastic-baggie free (see the Lunchbox Challenge). It was one easy way he felt that we could make a tangible difference. This simple goal led my kids to choose fresh, whole foods over anything that arrived in a box, bag, cup, or carton. We took it one step further by remaking some of our boxed favorites in a healthy way, like Power Bars (page 274) and Bitty Bites (page 221).

3. Cook Together
   For my kids, one of the keys to getting them to eat their lunches was to get them involved in making their own lunches. I know what you're thinking: "I barely have

enough time to get myself ready on busy mornings." I'm with you. But a bit of investment up front will save you time in the end. Start with making a meal plan each week for your lunches. Giving your kids responsibility for their choices helps you avoid nagging complaints like, "Why did you pack [insert offending food here] in my lunch? It gets mushy and I don't like it!" If they put it on the menu, and discover that they don't like it, they'll take responsibility for not packing it again and stop pointing the finger at you. Second, you start the week with a plan in place so you don't end up spending a hazy twenty minutes staring into the fridge wondering what to pack (again). Beyond planning, inviting kids to prepare their lunches makes an even bigger impact. On Sunday afternoon, set aside twenty minutes to wash, peel, and chop your fresh fruits and veggies for the week. Ready to take it a step further? Cook your Sunday dinner together and make enough for leftovers that can make another appearance as lunch in the week ahead.

The Lunchbox Challenge

At school, I learned that each person makes about seven pounds of trash every day. That trash usually ends up in our oceans and can hurt the animals. I challenge you to build a zero-waste lunchbox. Go through your lunchbox and count the number of things that can be reused, recycled, repurposed, terracycled, or composted. Then count the items that are trash or landfill. Make a graph of what you find. You'll be surprised to see how much trash you produce! Reduce the trash in your lunchbox each week, until you get to zero.

—JAMES LEE, AGE 7

A special note of thanks to James' teacher, Heather Connolly, for helping him discover that small changes can make a big impact—and that every person, no matter their age, can make a difference.

Leeks

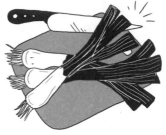

White might not be the first color you think of when eating your colors, but it is an important one to include in your diet. That's where leeks, garlic, and onions take center stage. All three of these ingredients are part of the lily family.[1] Their sulfur compounds, which can give rise to teary eyes, are the main source of their health benefits, which include fighting off cold and flu viruses.[2] For all of these reasons, I wanted to bring leeks to our table. But the lesson I learned from leeks remains a shining example of what *not* to do in your 52 New Foods Challenge.

The first misstep I made was deciding, without involving my kids, that we would try leeks. I didn't have time for shopping together, so I just grabbed a bundle of leeks from the shelf at our local market and figured I could convince everyone it was a good idea. I made the recipe when my kids were at school. "I'm too busy to involve the kids" was my crooked logic. The situation was made worse by overblending the potatoes until my leek soup looked like oobleck. I decided to serve it anyway. My husband, Anthony, said gently, "I think you need to try this one again." My kids outright refused to try it.

To avoid the mistakes I made, do three simple things. Always put your kids in charge of your adventure—let them choose your food each week. Then cook together. If I had at least prepared the leek soup with my kids, savoring each step of the way, I could rest knowing that the experience of cooking together was reward enough. As for recipe failures, let them roll off like water on a duck's back. Show your kids that failing is part of the journey, and we need to take it all in stride.

Make It a Game: 15 points
Eat Your Colors: White

> ### Invite Exploration
> "What other vegetables could we add to change the flavor of our soup?"

Healthy Leek Soup

Easy enough for a five-year-old to make, this healthy leek soup is a delicious addition to your 52 New Foods Challenge. Just be sure to cook it *with* your kids, not *for* your kids.

PREP TIME: 15 minutes

COOK TIME: 30 to 35 minutes

Serves 6

INGREDIENTS:

4 large leeks

4 russet potatoes

2 tablespoons unsalted butter

2½ cups Chicken Broth (page 99)

1 teaspoon kosher salt

2 cups nonfat milk

Minced chives, for garnish (optional)

Cook Together

Beginners: Give the leeks a bath. Peel the potatoes.

Experts: Chop the vegetables.

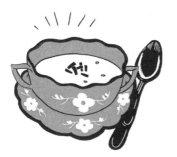

DIRECTIONS:

1 Chop the leeks into ½-inch pieces and clean them thoroughly (see How to Clean Leeks on page 148).

2 Peel the potatoes and chop them into ½-inch dice.

3 In a medium stockpot, melt the butter over medium heat. Add the leeks and sauté lightly for about 5 minutes, or until golden brown and fragrant.

4 Add the potatoes, broth, and salt to the leeks. Bring to a boil, then reduce the heat to maintain a simmer and cook for 25 to 30 minutes, until the potatoes are tender.

5 Let cool slightly, then carefully transfer the soup to a blender. Pulse gently until just combined. It's okay if there are a few chunks of leeks and potatoes remaining. (Be careful when blending hot liquids.)

Keep Trying Invite your kids to add something special to the recipe to make it unique, like fresh herbs from your window box garden or a new vegetable you discover at the local market. Parsnips, butternut squash, or sorrel all make wonderful additions.

Buy in Season Look for different varieties of leeks at your farmers' market, including King Richard, American Flag, and Pancho. Ask your kids to decipher the differences.

6 Return the soup to the pot and add the milk. Stir gently. Simmer over medium-low heat for 2 minutes more, until the soup is heated through.

7 Garnish with fresh chives. Serve warm.

Tip *Do not overblend. Overblending the soup was the reason my first version of this recipe turned into oobleck.*

Roasted Leeks

Roasting mellows the flavor of leeks (even further) and is another easy way to experiment with this wonderful "white" vegetable. We love this dish paired with Simple Sautéed Chicken (page 283) for a quick and delicious weeknight dinner.

PREP TIME: 10 minutes

COOK TIME: 15 minutes

Serves 4

INGREDIENTS:

4 large leeks

2 tablespoons extra-virgin olive oil

½ teaspoon kosher salt

DIRECTIONS:

1 Preheat the oven to 425°F.

2 Chop the leeks into ½-inch pieces and clean them thoroughly (see below).

3 On a rimmed baking sheet, toss the leeks with the oil and salt. Roast, turning several times, for 10 to 15 minutes, or until the leeks are crispy on the edges.

4 Serve immediately.

How to Clean Leeks

Because they are grown in sandy soil, leeks can be dirty. To clean them, follow these easy steps:

1. Chop off the root end and dark green tops of the leeks and discard. Cut the remaining white and light green portion in half lengthwise, then chop the leeks into ½-inch pieces.
2. Place the leeks in a large bowl of cold water. Separate the layers with your fingertips. Set aside for a few minutes. The dirt will sink to the bottom of the bowl while the leeks float to the top of the water.
3. Skim off the leeks into a sieve, then rinse again under cold water.

Avocados

When James began to explore his first foods, avocado starred at the top of his list. Packed with healthy fats, avocado is an excellent food for babies (and adults, too). He would eat mashed-up avocado like it was candy. I nurtured his love of this simple fruit, slicing it and offering it to him in the shell—the perfect bowl for his little hands. Catherine, on the other hand, would steer clear of any and all contact. Not knowing any better at the time, I let Catherine continue with her avoidance strategies. But by avoiding avocado, I was simply feeding Catherine's fear.

I needed to slowly start working to build that trust of new foods, even if it meant simply cooking something together without her trying it. So we started experimenting, first with making our own guacamole, which was great fun to mix and mash (even though she wouldn't try it). Then we moved to featuring this green fruit on our DIY sushi bar. Again, she remained reluctant, but the more avocado showed up at the table, the less fearful she became. When we decided to experiment with chocolate pudding made with a base of avocado, Catherine was skeptical (as was I) but was willing to give it a try. The result was a huge surprise: She liked it!

Avoiding any one food altogether does nothing to help build a healthy relationship with food as a whole. Your child might not ever get to the place where she likes avocado, and that's fine, but you need to keep trying. Avoiding the dragon will only get in the way of moving your family toward your goal.

Make It a Game: 10 points
Eat Your Colors: Green

Invite Exploration

"Why does avocado change its color when you open it?"

James' Guacamole

This simple guacamole recipe is easy for young children to make with very little assistance, and provided Catherine with a way to get to know avocado. Slicing the checkerboard pattern and scooping the cubes was her favorite part. It can be enjoyed as an accompaniment to quesadillas or chicken, or as a dip with fresh veggies. It's also great paired with Black Bean Burritos (page 172).

PREP TIME: 5 minutes

COOK TIME: 0 minutes

Makes about 3 cups

INGREDIENTS:

3 large avocados, preferably Hass

½ medium white onion, finely chopped

1 clove garlic, minced

1 tablespoon fresh lemon juice (from 1/2 lemon)

1 tablespoon fresh lime juice (from 1 lime)

Kosher salt

DIRECTIONS:

1   Halve the avocados and remove the pits. Using a paring knife, cut a checkerboard pattern into the flesh of the fruit, without cutting through the skin, slicing the avocado into small chunks.

2   Using a spoon, scoop around the fruit, between the flesh and the skin, to remove the cubes. (James likes to simply squeeze the flesh out of the skin into the bowl.)

3   In a medium bowl, use a potato masher to mash together the avocado, onion, garlic, lemon juice, and lime juice. Season with kosher salt to taste.

4   Serve immediately. Cover tightly with plastic wrap, pressed directly against the surface to prevent oxidation, if you plan to serve it later.

Tip Try your guacamole a couple of different ways. Go easy on the mashing and try it on the chunky side. Then try a smoother texture. Let your kids decide which way they prefer. You can also experiment by adding a few additional ingredients—bacon, tomatoes, or chile peppers—to make your own mix.

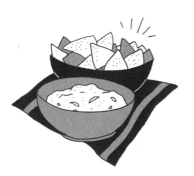

Cook Together

Beginners: Scoop out the avocado. Squeeze the lemons and limes. Mash the guacamole.

Experts: Slice the avocado. Chop the vegetables.

Avocado and Brown Rice Rolls

This recipe is fun for a DIY dinner. At our table, each person makes their own special roll, then we share. Add more color by including thinly sliced carrots, daikon radish, or cucumber along with the avocado.

PREP TIME: 15 minutes

COOK TIME: 0 minutes

Serves 4

INGREDIENTS:

3 cups cooked short-grain brown rice

2 tablespoons rice vinegar

1 tablespoon sugar

1 large Hass avocado

4 nori sheets (seaweed)

DIRECTIONS:

1 In a large wooden bowl, combine the rice, vinegar, and sugar. If the rice is just-cooked, let it cool slightly, for about 15 minutes, before rolling the sushi.

2 While the rice is cooling, prepare the avocado. Halve the avocados and remove the pits. Using a paring knife, slice the fruit into ½-inch-thick wedges without cutting through the skin. Using a spoon, scoop around the fruit, between the flesh and the skin, to remove the slices.

3 Place a large sheet of seaweed on a wooden sushi mat. Using your fingers, press a handful of rice onto the seaweed and spread it into an even layer. The rice should cover about half of the sheet. One inch from the edge closest to you, add a few slices of avocado in a single layer.

4 Starting from the side closest to you, roll the sushi into a pinwheel. Squeeze gently and lift the mat away as you go. Transfer the roll to a cutting board and slice it into 6 to 8 pieces. Repeat with the remaining ingredients.

The Chocolate Rocket

This sweet treat was such a surprise at our family table. Like Catherine, I was skeptical that I would like the taste of avocado in a pudding. But the texture was so smooth and the combination of flavors so delicious that it won us over. Just remember not to *sneak* in any ingredients. Have your kids make this recipe, so they know what's in the food they're eating.

PREP TIME: 10 minutes

COOK TIME: 0 minutes

Serves 8

INGREDIENTS:

2 medium Hass avocados

½ cup unsweetened cocoa powder

½ cup light brown sugar

⅓ cup nonfat milk

2 teaspoons pure vanilla extract

Whipped cream and fresh fruit, for serving

DIRECTIONS:

1 Halve the avocados and remove the pits. Using a spoon, scoop around the fruit, between the flesh and the skin, to remove the flesh. Place it in a food processor fitted with the metal blade.

2 Add the cocoa powder, sugar, milk, and vanilla and process for 2 minutes, or until smooth and no chunks of avocado remain.

3 Chill for 10 minutes.

4 Serve in small cups with a dollop of whipped cream. Top with fresh fruit.

Keep Trying Serve your avocado lots of different ways: as a dip, loaded into a burrito or layered on a sandwich, or eaten straight from the shell.

Satsuma Mandarin Oranges

Like bouncing balls on a playground, mandarin oranges at the market add cheerful pops of color to dreary winter days and herald the coming of Chinese New Year. Nature's perfect "fast food," mandarin oranges are regularly featured as lunchbox treats, after-school snacks, and even dessert for my family during the bleak winter months. With friends like these, who needs vitamin C supplements?

You may be thinking, "My kids already like oranges. It's not a new food!" But consider this: Oranges may not be a "challenging" food for your kids but they are a key to the more challenging foods to come. For many families, oranges fall into the safety zone, along with apples and carrots, relied on by parents of picky eaters as one of the only sources of color their kids will eat. Oranges also provide an easy way to start cooking together. The fun of peeling, squeezing, freezing, and blending this juicy fruit is contagious!

What has helped my kids become more willing to try new foods in general is getting into the habit of trying their favorite foods, like mandarin oranges, in lots of different ways, and making the recipes together so that they can feel ownership in what we make. That kind of safe experimentation builds confidence and fosters creativity, which translates into my kids viewing themselves as people who like to cook and try new things. That positive self-image may start at the family table, but it extends into other aspects of their lives as well.

Make It a Game: 5 points
Eat Your Colors: Yellow/Orange

Invite Exploration

"What new ways could we try mandarin oranges?"

"What do you notice that's different about mandarin oranges compared to other kinds of oranges?"

Easy Satsuma Granita

This easy granita recipe was a fun project for my kids and me! It is a simple twist on a favorite winter fruit, and a healthy alternative for dessert. If your family is like ours, you don't have time to scrape, then freeze, then scrape, then freeze, to create a granita. Instead, we made our granita the easy way, with our food processor. We tried the recipe two ways: one with clementine and the other with Satsumas. The Satsumas were far superior, both in color and taste, so we'd highly recommend hunting them down for this recipe. It will be well worth your effort!

PREP TIME: 5 minutes

WAIT TIME: 90 to 120 minutes

Serves 4

INGREDIENTS:

8 Satsuma mandarin oranges

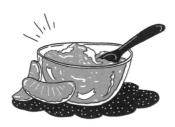

DIRECTIONS:

1 Slice the oranges in half, cutting through the middle of the orange as opposed to top to bottom. Using a simple citrus press, squeeze the juice out of the oranges.

2 Pour the juice into an ice cube tray and place it in the freezer. It can take up to 2 hours for the juice to freeze completely.

3 Once frozen, remove the juice cubes from the tray and load them into a food processor.

4 Pulse until the frozen juice looks like slush.

5 Serve immediately.

Cook Together

Beginners: Squeeze the oranges. Pour the juice.

Experts: Slice the oranges.

Tip: Squeezing is the best part of this recipe for my kids! Set up on a rimmed baking sheet to contain the mess.

Orange and Fennel Salad

This simple orange salad is super flexible. It's easy to prepare and can be made ahead. When time is tight and I need to add another color to our table, I pull out this salad. It's also great packed in a lunchbox. If your kids are slow to warm to the flavor of fennel, substitute chopped celery.

PREP TIME: 10 minutes

COOK TIME: 0 minutes

Serves 4

INGREDIENTS:

2 cups sliced Satsuma mandarin orange segments (from about 6 oranges)

½ cup thinly sliced fennel

1 teaspoon coarsely chopped fresh mint

1 tablespoon extra-virgin olive oil

1 tablespoon fresh lemon juice (from ½ lemon)

Kosher salt

DIRECTIONS:

1 In a medium bowl, combine the oranges, fennel, and mint. Drizzle with the oil and lemon juice. Toss gently to combine. Add kosher salt to taste.

2 Store, covered, in the refrigerator for up to 1 week.

Buy in Season If you're nice, Santa will pop a mandarin orange in your stocking for good luck.

Orange Dippers

This is a favorite recipe for my kids at Valentine's Day. It makes a pretty, edible bouquet. If you're feeling fancy, dip the end of the chocolate-covered oranges in a few sprinkles.

PREP TIME: 10 minutes

COOK TIME: 30 minutes

Serves 4

INGREDIENTS:

6 Satsuma mandarin oranges

½ cup dark chocolate chips

Vegetable oil (optional)

DIRECTIONS:

1 Peel and segment the oranges. Place each orange wedge on the end of a wooden skewer. Set aside on a large rimmed baking sheet lined with parchment.

2 In a large saucepan, bring 2 cups water to a simmer. Remove from the heat, then place the chocolate in a heatproof bowl and set it over the heated water. Stir gently. You can add a bit of vegetable oil to the chocolate to make it easier to work with.

3 When the chocolate is just melted, dip the edge of each orange segment into the chocolate and swirl gently. Place the skewers back on the baking sheet to cool.

4 Serve in a vase, like a flower arrangement.

Grapefruits

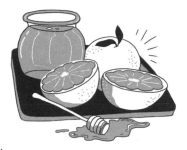

Sour gummy bears. I'm not proud of it, but those words describe the only sour food (though technically not a food) that my son, James, will eat. Like me, he has a bit of a sweet tooth. So it should come as no surprise that whenever grapefruit showed up on our table, he'd dodge it with the nimbleness of a ninja. The sour flavor on his tongue literally made his whole face pucker. That is, until broiling entered the picture.

Broiling grapefruit completely changes its flavor. In the same way that garlic goes from sharp to mellow when roasted, grapefruit transforms from lip-puckering sour to lip-smacking sweet. The smell is beautiful, too. The morning I popped the grapefruit in the oven, it was only a few minutes before I heard the pitter-patter of feet coming down the stairs and voices inquiring, "What are you making for breakfast today?" My kitchen smelled like a fancy boutique.

Smoothing out grapefruit's sour notes was definitely a step in the right direction. It was the only way to get James to try it. But it's still not on his list of favorite foods. So instead, when the gray winter months need a burst of freshness, I invite James to squeeze the grapefruit for recipes that call for its juice, slice it up and drizzle it with honey when we're having it for breakfast, or just marvel at the beautiful pattern its flesh reveals (yes, another Fibonacci sequence, if you count carefully). I do this knowing that it's not important that he doesn't like grapefruit, but what's most important is that he's willing to keep trying, and that we cook together, which is really what it's all about.

Make It a Game: 5 points
Eat Your Colors: Red or Yellow/Orange

> ### Invite Exploration
> "I wonder why the flavor of grapefruit changes so dramatically when it is baked?"

Broiled Grapefruit

Delicately dressed with a touch of honey and a sprinkle of cinnamon and ginger, broiled grapefruit is a quick and tasty breakfast treat.

PREP TIME: 2 minutes

COOK TIME: 3 to 5 minutes

Serves 4

INGREDIENTS:

2 grapefruits, halved

2 teaspoons honey

Ground cinnamon

Ground ginger

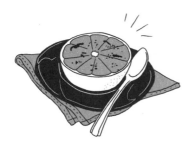

DIRECTIONS:

1   Preheat the oven to broil. Line a rimmed baking sheet with foil or parchment paper.

2   Wash the grapefruit and cut it in half through the middle. Using a small paring knife, cut around the outside of the grapefruit and then slice along the edge of each of its segments to loosen the fruit. Place the halves cut-side up on the lined baking sheet.

3   Top each grapefruit half with ½ teaspoon of the honey, spreading gently over the fruit with the back of a spoon. Sprinkle each half lightly with cinnamon and ginger.

4   Broil for 3 to 5 minutes, or until tops are slightly browned but not burned.

5   Serve immediately.

Cook Together

Beginners: Spread the honey. Sprinkle the spices.

Experts: Slice and segment the grapefruits.

Grapefruit and Mint Dressing

This simple dressing makes a refreshing and light dip. Although my kids aren't fans of salad, they are willing to try dipping butter lettuce leaves and fresh-cut veggies in this dressing.

PREP TIME: 10 minutes

COOK TIME: 0 minutes

Makes ¾ cup

INGREDIENTS:

½ cup fresh grapefruit juice (from 1 medium grapefruit)

¼ cup extra-virgin olive oil

1 tablespoon coarsely chopped fresh mint

½ teaspoon kosher salt

DIRECTIONS:

1 In a medium bowl or salad dressing shaker, combine the grapefruit juice, oil, mint, and salt. Mix or shake thoroughly to combine.

2 Serve in small bowls with lettuce leaves or freshly cut veggies for dipping.

Avocado and Grapefruit Boats

This is a great way to pair two new foods together. If your kids have not yet warmed up to the flavor of avocado, serve the grapefruit salad on its own.

PREP TIME: 10 minutes

COOK TIME: 0 minutes

Serves 4

INGREDIENTS:

1 tablespoon extra-virgin olive oil

1 tablespoon fresh lime juice (from ½ lime)

¼ teaspoon kosher salt

1 large grapefruit

2 large Hass avocados

Fresh mint leaves, for garnish

DIRECTIONS:

1 In a small bowl, whisk together the oil, lime juice, and salt.

2 Peel and slice the grapefruit into ½-inch pieces. Add them to the bowl with the dressing and toss thoroughly to combine. Set aside.

3 Slice the avocados in half and remove the pits. Leaving the skin intact, use a paring knife to cut a checkerboard pattern in the flesh of the fruit, without cutting through the skin, slicing the avocado into small chunks.

4 Place the avocado halves cut-side up on a small platter. Portion the grapefruit mixture evenly into each boat.

5 Drizzle with any remaining lime dressing from the bowl. Garnish with mint. Serve immediately.

Keep Trying Pour any remaining grapefruit juice into an ice cube tray. Cover with plastic wrap, then poke toothpicks through the wrap into each square. Freeze overnight. Remove the plastic wrap and enjoy your mini grapefruit pops. It's another easy and fun way to try grapefruit.

Kumquats

Chinese New Year is the centerpiece of celebrations for my Chinese family. Different foods play specific roles in preparing for the year ahead, but kumquats have a particularly special meaning. Translated, their Chinese name means "gold orange," which is telling—they symbolize prosperity. In January, you'll begin to notice small evergreen trees with bright pops of orange, sometimes adorned with red "lucky money" envelopes, at Chinese markets, restaurants, and homes throughout your neighborhood. If the folklore is true, they will bring good fortune to those families.

So to celebrate the start of the Lunar New Year, we decided to experiment with kumquats. Eyes widened at the table when I told the story of how kumquats are thought to bring good things to families who grow and eat them—that made them even more intriguing, and worth a try. Who wouldn't want to have a hand in bringing good fortune?

For such a small fruit, they pack a surprisingly big flavor punch. We tried two varieties—the oval-shaped Nagami, which is more tart, and the rounded Marumi, which is more sweet. We sampled the fruit straight from the vine and then simmered them down into a sweet jam. They are also delicious sliced and tossed into a salad or bowl of green beans—the contrast of color between the orange and green is beautifully striking.

Make It a Game: 5 points
Eat Your Colors: Yellow/Orange

Invite Exploration

"I wonder why kumquats and mandarin oranges signify prosperity in China? Could they mean something different in other cultures?"

Good Luck Jam

This sweet jam made with kumquats and honey adds a simple citrus touch to savory dishes: a burst of sunshine and prosperity to start the New Year! We appreciated how easy this recipe was to make, since you can skip the jars that are typically involved in making a jam if you eat it within a week. This tasty spread is wonderful paired with cheese, bread, or savory dishes, like Easy Roasted Chicken (page 282) and Sesame-Crusted Salmon (page 224). My kids love eating it, for good luck!

PREP TIME: 5 minutes

COOK TIME: 15 to 20 minutes

Makes about 1 cup

INGREDIENTS:

2 cups kumquats

½ cup honey

DIRECTIONS:

1   Wash the kumquats and cut them into quarters. Remove the seeds. See if you can spot a Fibonacci sequence inside (see page 138).

2   In a small saucepan, bring ½ cup water to a boil. Add the honey, then reduce the heat to maintain a simmer and cook for 3 to 4 minutes, or until a thin syrup forms.

3   Add the kumquats to the syrup and simmer gently for 10 minutes. Remove and discard any remaining seeds that float to the top.

4   Over a large bowl, drain the kumquats through a sieve and set aside to cool. Return the syrup to the pot and simmer gently for 3 to 5 minutes.

5   To serve, drizzle the reduced syrup over the cooked kumquats. This dish can be served warm or cold. Store in a glass container in the refrigerator for up to 1 week.

Cook Together

Beginners: Remove the seeds. Combine the ingredients. Stir the pot. Drizzle!

Experts: Cut the fruit.

Kumquat Salad

This colorful salad is an easy way to feature kumquats on your table. Pairing them with a Gateway Food—green beans—makes it easier for your kids to give kumquats a try.

PREP TIME: 10 minutes

COOK TIME: 5 to 7 minutes

Serves 4

INGREDIENTS:

1 pound green beans, trimmed and cut into 2-inch pieces

1 cup kumquats, thinly sliced and seeded

1 tablespoon extra-virgin olive oil

¼ teaspoon kosher salt

DIRECTIONS:

1 In a medium saucepan, bring 2 inches of water to a boil. Place the green beans in a steamer insert and set them over the boiling water. Cook the beans for 5 to 7 minutes, or until they are bright green and tender when pierced with a fork. Steam them a little less if you prefer your beans on the crunchy side. Drain the beans and give them a bath in a large bowl of ice water to bring back their color. Drain again and place in a large bowl.

2 Add the kumquat slices, oil, and salt to the beans. Toss to combine.

3 Serve immediately.

Buy in Season Head out to your local Chinatown or Chinese market and pick up a basket of fresh kumquats. Ask the farmer or shopkeeper how they include this seasonal fruit in their Chinese New Year celebrations.

Grow It Kumquat trees are hardy and compact, making them perfect for container gardens in the winter months.

Keep Trying In the end, my kids had the most fun eating the fruit straight from the vine. Sometimes, simple is best!

Asian Pears

When my kids spotted Asian pears at the market and decided to make them our new food of the week, we spent some time exploring different dishes we could make together—salads, soups, and sauces. Sauces! Maybe a new twist on an old favorite—applesauce? Like most families, applesauce was a staple in our fridge when my kids were toddlers. Week after week, I would religiously buy those little plastic cups filled with sauce in the hope that I would be saved from snack-time meltdowns.

When we set out to make our own version of applesauce, I figured it would be a one-timer. Why would I make it when it was so easy to buy it in a perfectly portioned cup? But in the same way that it was easy to buy applesauce, it was (surprisingly) easy to make applesauce—or Asian pear sauce, in this case. There was lots of peeling. It kept Catherine and James happily occupied for at least twenty minutes—time I would never invest in peeling by myself. Then there was the mashing, yet another job that my kids loved.

As our sauce simmered in the pot, their excitement grew, and they were rewarded with a deliciously warm and satisfying treat. Satisfying not only because of the healthy ingredients but also because of the pleasure that comes from eating and sharing a dish you have made with your own hands. Enjoying our snack with my kids, I thought, *This was easier than I expected.* And the rewards were much greater than anything that could be packed in a plastic cup.

Make It a Game: 5 points
Eat Your Colors: Yellow/Orange

Invite Exploration

"What combination of foods do you think an Asian pear tastes like?"

Easy Asian Pear Sauce

Pear sauce made with crisp Asian pears and a hint of ginger is an easy and fun twist on homemade applesauce. It's perfect paired with Gigi's Roasted Pork Tenderloin (page 286).

PREP TIME: 20 minutes

COOK TIME: 25 to 30 minutes

Makes about 6 cups

INGREDIENTS:

2 pounds Asian pears

2 pounds Fuji apples

3 tablespoons lemon juice (from 1½ lemons)

1 tablespoon finely chopped peeled fresh ginger

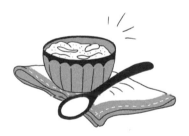

DIRECTIONS:

1 Using a potato peeler, remove the skins from the pears and apples. Core them and chop the fruit into ¼-inch pieces.

2 In a large stockpot, combine the pears, apples, lemon juice, ginger, and 1½ cups water. Bring to a boil, then reduce the heat to maintain a simmer and cook for 25 to 30 minutes, or until the fruit is soft. The Asian pears will remain slightly crunchy compared to the apples.

3 Remove the pot from the heat and let the mixture cool. Invite your kids to mash the fruit mixture with a potato masher until you achieve the texture you prefer. This can easily be done in the pot once it has cooled slightly. We left small chunks of pear in our sauce.

4 Serve warm or cold.

Cook Together

Beginners: Peel the fruit. Squeeze the juice. Mash the fruit.

Experts: Chop the fruit.

Catherine's Winter Fruit Salad

My daughter, Catherine, loves the peeling and chopping in this simple recipe. For beginners, focus on the peeling. For more advanced cooks, let them do the chopping. Invite everyone to add their favorite fruit to the mix to make the recipe unique.

PREP TIME: 15 minutes

COOK TIME: 0 minutes

Makes 2 cups

INGREDIENTS:

1 large Asian pear, peeled, cored, and cut into ½-inch pieces

1 medium orange, peeled and cut into ½-inch pieces

½ cup pomegranate seeds (see box on page 115)

1 tablespoon fresh lemon juice (from ½ lemon)

DIRECTIONS:

In a large bowl, combine the pear, orange, and pomegranate seeds. Add the lemon juice and toss to combine.

Keep Trying For variety, substitute apples in your favorite recipes with Asian pears.

Quinoa

What is it with white? Even after months of working on eating colorful meals, if I take my eyes off the course, white—plain pasta and rice—becomes our default.

My strategy hasn't been to fight against it tirelessly—banishing white rice and pasta from our table would only lead to my crew abandoning ship. Instead, I use the Work-Your-Way-Up Strategy (see page 56) to add healthier alternatives when I can to nudge us (slowly) in the right direction. Quinoa is one of those alternatives.

Though it serves the same purpose on our plates as pasta and rice, quinoa is a whole lot better for us than plain ol' white. Calorie for calorie, it's got more protein than brown rice (another nutritional rock star when it comes to competing with whites).[3] The trick is making it taste better than sawdust. I want to like quinoa because of its heightened nutritional profile, but I find it rather unfulfilling in the taste department.

So we started to experiment. Like most of the other foods we tried, I found quinoa was much more welcome at our table when we cooked it together. Over the holidays, we dolled up a batch of quinoa with apples, sweet potato, walnuts, and maple syrup to make an alternative to stuffing for our turkey. The combination of sweet and nutty flavors was a huge hit. But our favorite cooking project was fashioning those little grains into miniature savory cakes. Not only because it was great fun for my kids to get their hands in the mix making mini patties, but those hot cakes were tasty and satisfying and made us forget, for one brief moment, about white.

Make It a Game: 5 points
Eat Your Colors: Healthy Grains

> ### Invite Exploration
>
> "What other ingredients could we add to our Quinoa Crumble Cakes?"
>
> "How else could we make a recipe with these ingredients?"

Quinoa Crumble Cakes

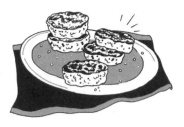

This recipe is great fun to cook together. My kids love mixing the ingredients and forming the cakes with their hands, just like play clay.

PREP TIME: 15 minutes

COOK TIME: about 20 minutes

Serves 4

INGREDIENTS:

2½ cups cooked quinoa (see Basic Quinoa, page 169)

4 large eggs, beaten

1 cup whole wheat bread crumbs

½ cup grated Parmesan cheese

1 medium apple, finely chopped (about ½ cup)

½ medium onion, finely chopped (about ¼ cup)

½ teaspoon kosher salt

Extra-virgin olive oil

DIRECTIONS:

1　In a large bowl, combine the cooked quinoa and eggs.

2　Add the bread crumbs, Parmesan, apples, onion, and salt to the quinoa mixture. Encourage your kids to grease their hands with olive oil, then combine the ingredients pressing firmly, until a handful of the mixture easily forms into a ball. The oil will prevent the mixture from sticking to their fingers. If it falls apart too easily, add a touch of water.

3　Craft the quinoa mixture into small cakes, about the size of your child's palm. You should end up with between 12 and 14 cakes.

4　Heat a large frying pan over medium-low heat, then add 2 tablespoons of oil (or enough to coat the pan evenly). Add half of the cakes and cook for 5 to 7 minutes, or until the bottoms are golden brown and crispy. Using a spatula,

Cook Together

Beginners: Mix the ingredients. Mold the cakes.

Experts: Chop the apples and onion. Fry the cakes.

Keep Trying The first time we made Quinoa Crumble Cakes, the flavor was a little strong for Catherine, so we swapped out the onions for apples. Equally delicious. Just be sure to dice the apples into small pieces to avoid the cakes falling apart in the pan. You can also use the Work-Your-Way-Up Strategy (see page 56) with this dish. Start with more diced apple than onion. After a few tries, slowly increase the proportion of onions to apples until you find the right mix for your family.

flip the patties and cook the other side for 5 to 7 minutes more.

5 Repeat with the remaining quinoa patties, refreshing the oil between batches.

6 Cool the cakes on a plate lined with paper towels before serving.

Recipe inspired by one of my favorite chefs, Heidi Swanson, author of Super Natural Every Day.

Basic Quinoa

Make a big batch of quinoa on Sunday and store it in a glass container in your fridge. It's a huge time saver on busy weeknights.

PREP TIME: 5 minutes
COOK TIME: 20 minutes
Makes 2½ to 3 cups

INGREDIENTS:

1 cup quinoa
2 cups Chicken Broth (page 99)
¼ teaspoon kosher salt

DIRECTIONS:

1 In a small saucepan, combine the quinoa with the broth and salt.

2 Cover, bring to a boil over medium heat, then reduce the heat to low and simmer for 15 to 20 minutes, or until the liquid has been absorbed and the grains are tender and fluffy.

3 Serve immediately, or let cool, then store in a glass container in the refrigerator for up to 1 week. This recipe should yield 2½ to 3 cups of cooked quinoa.

Tip *You can also make quinoa in your rice cooker. Just stick to a 2:1 liquid-to-grain ratio.*

Quinoa Stuffing with Apple, Sweet Potato, and Walnuts

This recipe is a delicious alternative to bread stuffing. It feels fancy enough to feature at your holiday table, but it's easy enough to make on a weeknight.

PREP TIME: 20 minutes

COOK TIME: 40 minutes

Serves 4

INGREDIENTS:

2 large Braeburn apples

2 large orange-fleshed sweet potatoes

2 tablespoons extra-virgin olive oil

1 tablespoon fresh lemon juice (from ½ lemon)

¼ cup maple syrup

¼ teaspoon ground ginger

¼ teaspoon ground cinnamon

3 cups Basic Quinoa (page 169)

1 cup coarsely chopped walnuts

Handful of fresh parsley leaves

Kosher salt

DIRECTIONS:

1 Preheat the oven to 400°F.

2 Peel, core, and chop the apples into ½-inch pieces. Peel and chop the potatoes into ½-inch pieces.

3 In a large baking dish, combine the apples and potatoes with the oil, lemon juice, maple syrup, ginger, and cinnamon. Bake, turning occasionally, for 35 to 40 minutes, or until the potatoes are tender when pierced with a fork.

4 Add the quinoa, walnuts, and parsley to the baked apples and potatoes. Stir to combine. Season with kosher salt to taste.

5 Serve immediately.

Recipe inspired by my food friend and fellow mom Marla Meridith of Family Fresh Cooking.

Black Beans

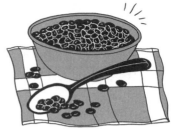

During our 52 New Foods Challenge, we became a picky family. Not picky in terms of *which* foods we would eat, but picky in terms of *how* those foods came to our table. In getting to know our local farmers, and the foods they worked so hard to grow, we began to learn firsthand why organic makes a difference. We were slowly beginning to realize that our food choices made an impact beyond our dinner table. The problem was this: Choosing to eat organic can be costly.

So I started to concoct a plan for how to eat organic, without eating away too much of our bank account. Beans played a major role in that plan. Not only are beans nutritionally sound, they are cheap and plentiful. Compared to an organic whole chicken, beans are a bargain. As with most things on this adventure, I needed to spend some time getting educated. Aside from the kidney beans that my gram worked into her minestrone soup, I had very little exposure to cooking with beans of any kind. Black beans were one of my son James' favorite foods, but one that we rarely enjoyed at home, so we decided to start there.

I was overjoyed to learn that beans can be prepared in a slow cooker. It's so easy that I can barely call it cooking. It saved me time and allowed us to cook up a batch big enough that we could use beans in various dishes throughout the week (while saving a few beans). Our current favorite recipe is Black Bean Soup (page 174). Try featuring beans as the main dish on your menu at least once a week—they are an easy, low-cost option for Meatless Monday.

Make It a Game: 10 points
Eat Your Colors: Protein

Invite Exploration

"Which ingredients that we haven't tried can we add to our Black Bean Burritos?"

Black Bean Burritos

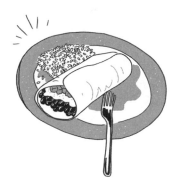

Black Bean Burritos are an easy weeknight dinner option and a great way to go meatless one night a week. We like to set up this recipe DIY style, so everyone can make their own mix.

PREP TIME: 5 minutes

COOK TIME: 10 minutes

Serves 6

INGREDIENTS:

6 large whole wheat tortillas

1½ cups shredded cheddar cheese

1½ cups cooked brown rice

1½ cups Basic Black Beans (page 173)

1 large avocado, sliced into ½-inch-thick wedges

¾ cup chopped tomatoes

Cook Together

Beginners: Sort the beans. Assemble the burritos.

Experts: Slice the avocado. Chop the tomatoes.

DIRECTIONS:

1 In a large sauté pan, warm each tortilla over medium heat for 1 to 2 minutes, or until small bubbles appear. Flip the tortilla, turn down the heat, and add ¼ cup of the shredded cheddar cheese. Warm for 1 to 2 minutes more. Slide the tortilla out of the pan onto a wooden cutting board.

2 Add ¼ cup of the rice, ¼ cup of the beans, a few avocado slices, and 2 tablespoons of the tomatoes to the center of each tortilla.

3 Fold in the bottom and top edges of the tortilla over the rice and beans, then roll the tortilla up into a cylinder. Set it back in the pan over low heat to warm each side for 1 to 2 minutes.

4 Repeat for the remaining tortillas.

Tip To add more color, include thinly sliced jícama and carrot matchsticks, Garlic Corn (page 255), or shaved radicchio.

Tip Swap the rice for scrambled eggs and try these burritos for breakfast.

Keep Trying Encourage everyone to make one burrito for themselves and two to share. Then trade. That way everyone can try a taste of something new.

Basic Black Beans

A budget-friendly staple, black beans can be made ahead and stored in the refrigerator, making it easy to use them in various ways throughout the week.

PREP TIME: 12 hours

COOK TIME: 6 to 8 hours

Makes about 3 cups

INGREDIENTS:

1 (16-ounce) bag dried black beans

12 cups Chicken Broth (page 99) or water

1 tablespoon garlic powder

Kosher salt

DIRECTIONS:

1   Sort the black beans, removing any debris or broken beans. Place the beans in a bowl, add water to cover, and set aside to soak overnight. Be sure the water fully covers the beans.

2   Drain and rinse the beans, then place them in a slow cooker along with the broth and garlic powder. Stir to combine.

3   Set the slow cooker to low and cook the black beans for 6 hours, or until the beans are tender.

4   Season to taste with salt. Serve warm with a little bit of fresh corn and a sprig of parsley or mint for garnish. Or transfer to an airtight container and refrigerate for up to 1 week.

Tip *If you don't have a slow cooker, you can make this recipe in a stockpot. Bring the broth and beans to a boil, skimming the surface to remove the foam, then reduce the heat and simmer for 2 hours, or until the beans are tender but not splitting.*

Cook Together

Soaking the beans results in a flavor and texture that is much better than any beans we tasted from a can. It takes some planning, but it's worth the time investment.

Black Bean Soup

This hearty soup is one of James' favorites. Paired with Portobello Mushroom Quesadillas (page 198), it makes a quick weeknight meal. It's also great packed in a lunchbox.

PREP TIME: 15 minutes

COOK TIME: 15 minutes

Serves 4

INGREDIENTS:

2 tablespoons extra-virgin olive oil

1 medium onion, finely chopped

1 red bell pepper, seeded, cored, and chopped

½ teaspoon kosher salt

1 clove garlic, finely chopped

4 cups Chicken Broth (page 99)

3 cups Basic Black Beans (page 173)

Lime juice, for serving

Cilantro leaves, for garnish

DIRECTIONS:

1 Heat a large stockpot over medium-high heat. Add the oil, onion, pepper, and salt and sauté for 2 to 3 minutes, or until the onions soften and turn translucent. Add the garlic and cook for 1 minute more.

2 Add the broth and beans and bring to a boil. Reduce the heat to maintain a simmer and cook for 5 minutes, or until the soup thickens slightly and is warmed through.

3 Garnish with a squeeze of lime juice and a sprinkle of fresh cilantro leaves.

Tip *Before adding the beans and broth to the onion mixture, separate 1 cup of black beans and 1 cup of chicken broth and add it to the simmering vegetables. Puree the mixture with an immersion blender, until it forms a chunky paste. Then add the remaining chicken broth and beans and bring to a boil. My kids prefer this soup without the puree, but this is another variation you can try.*

Spring

Asparagus

Spears standing tall, asparagus lined up in crates at the farmers' market looks like boxes of fresh green crayons begging to color your table. The perennial harbingers of spring, asparagus is one of my favorite ways to welcome the start of Sunday brunch season! Despite its good looks and cheery nutritional profile (it's full of folate),[1] it was challenging to get my kids to try asparagus—the taste can be a tad on the bitter side for young palates. So I turned to one of my trusted new food vehicles: mini frittatas.

A simple Italian frittata, the smell of this dish simmering always transports me back to my gram's kitchen at Easter time. In addition to being a delicious brunch companion, this simple recipe has a few added benefits. For one, it's a fun way to cook together. The youngest members of your clan can crack and beat the eggs. More experienced chefs can chop the asparagus, potatoes, and onions. Everyone can be involved in the assembly, which is where this recipe sings. Second, it's a reliable new food vehicle (see page 57)—a gentle way to get your kids to try a new food. You can equally use this recipe as a way to introduce asparagus, kale, mushrooms, or broccoli.

Serve up your ingredients in small bowls and let each person make their own mix. More asparagus or less (but encourage them to give it a try). Onions or not. With cheese or without. Have each person make one for themselves and two to share. That way, everyone can have a no-brainer option to enjoy, and a few that are a little more challenging to try. When we made this dish, Catherine was skeptical about the asparagus, but James made one for her to try, so she obliged. To her surprise, she liked it!

Make It a Game: 15
Eat Your Colors: Green, White/Brown, or Blue/Purple

Invite Exploration

Let your kids personalize their frittatas by adding the amount and kind of vegetables that they feel is right for them. Encourage them to make a couple of variations to give different tastes (and new veggies) a try.

Mini Asparagus Frittata (aka Savory Muffins)

Baked with asparagus, onions, and eggs, this easy asparagus frittata recipe was a huge hit with my family. Catherine calls them Savory Muffins. The perfect size for little hands, these mini frittatas are great for a spring brunch. Plus, they're super portable, which makes them an easy addition to your healthy lunchbox.

PREP TIME: 10 minutes

COOK TIME: 30 minutes

Makes 12 muffins

INGREDIENTS:

2 tablespoons extra-virgin olive oil

½ large white onion, cut into ¼-inch pieces

1 medium red potato, cut into ¼-inch pieces

1 pound asparagus (about 1 bunch), trimmed and cut into ¼-inch pieces

10 large eggs

¼ teaspoon kosher salt

½ cup shredded mozzarella cheese

4 slices bacon, cooked and chopped (optional)

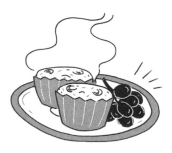

DIRECTIONS:

1 Preheat the oven to 350°F. Lightly spray a standard muffin tin with olive oil. For best results, use silicone baking cups in the pan.

2 Heat a medium frying pan over medium heat. Add the oil and onions and sauté for 2 to 3 minutes, until the onions are translucent and slightly browned. Add the potatoes and sauté for 3 to 4 minutes more. Finally, add the asparagus and mix together. Sauté for 3 to 4 minutes more. Set aside in a small bowl.

3 In a large bowl, beat together the eggs and salt.

4 Pour the egg mixture into the prepared baking cups, filling each cup about halfway. Add a spoonful of the cooked vegetables to each cup and sprinkle with mozzarella. Add the cooked bacon if using. Divide the

Cook Together

Beginners: Crack and beat the eggs. Snap the spears. Assemble the frittata.

Experts: Chop and sauté the vegetables.

Tip: Use a small measuring cup to portion the egg mixture into the muffin cups. This will make pouring easier for your kids.

remaining egg mixture among the cups, filling them almost all the way to the top.

5 Bake for 20 minutes, or until the tops spring back when lightly touched.

6 Serve immediately.

Tip For maximum flexibility, sauté each vegetable separately and transfer to small serving bowls before assembly. The downside is it takes a little longer to prep, but the upside is kids can more easily personalize their dish.

Roasted Asparagus

As your kids warm up to the flavor of asparagus, try it roasted! I love this recipe because it's so simple. My kids enjoy snapping the spears, then painting them with olive oil—a fun and easy way to get them involved. There is very little prep, and the asparagus cooks quickly, which makes this dish great for a weeknight.

PREP TIME: 5 minutes

COOK TIME: 10 minutes

Serves 4

INGREDIENTS:

1 bunch asparagus (about 1 pound)

1 tablespoon extra-virgin olive oil

¼ teaspoon kosher salt

Squeeze of fresh lemon juice

DIRECTIONS:

1 Preheat the oven to 450°F. Rinse the asparagus and then snap off the ends. Arrange the spears in a single, even layer on a rimmed baking sheet.

2 Using a pastry brush, paint the spears with the oil. Sprinkle with salt.

3 Roast for 10 minutes, or until the thick part of the spears can be easily pierced with a fork.

4 Add a squeeze of lemon before serving.

Tip To remove the tough ends of asparagus, invite your kids to simply bend gently near the base of the spear. It will snap off easily. No knives required!

Asparagus with Ginger-Soy Glaze

This is a delicious variation on roasted asparagus. The savory ginger-soy glaze is perfect for drizzling and dipping.

PREP TIME: 5 minutes

COOK TIME: 10 minutes

Serves 4

INGREDIENTS:

1 bunch asparagus (about 1 pound)

1 tablespoon extra-virgin olive oil

¼ teaspoon kosher salt

3 tablespoons tamari

1 tablespoon chopped peeled fresh ginger

1 tablespoon honey

DIRECTIONS:

1   Preheat the oven to 450°F. Rinse the asparagus and then snap off the ends. Arrange the spears in a single, even layer on a rimmed baking sheet.

2   Using a pastry brush, paint the spears with the oil. Sprinkle with salt.

3   Roast for 10 minutes, or until the thick part of the spears can be easily pierced with a fork.

4   While the asparagus is baking, in a small bowl, whisk together the tamari, ginger, and honey.

5   When the asparagus is done, use a pastry brush to paint the spears with half of the glaze and toss gently in the pan. Serve the remaining glaze on the side. Let your kids drizzle and dip!

Bow-Tie Pasta with Asparagus and Bacon

This simple pasta dish makes a quick weeknight dinner. If your kids resist mixing everything together in one dish, serve the ingredients in individual bowls and let everyone make their own mix. Like mini frittatas, this basic pasta dish is another reliable new-food vehicle.

PREP TIME: 10 minutes

COOK TIME: 15 minutes

Serves 4

INGREDIENTS:

1 pound whole wheat farfalle or penne (uncooked)

1 tablespoon extra-virgin olive oil

4 slices bacon, cut into ½-inch pieces

1 pound asparagus, trimmed and cut into 2-inch pieces

½ cup grated Parmesan cheese

2 tablespoons fresh lemon juice (from 1 lemon)

½ teaspoon kosher salt

DIRECTIONS:

1 Bring a large pot of salted water to a boil. Cook the pasta according to the package directions. Drain the pasta and reserve 1 cup of water from the pot. Set aside.

2 Return the pot to medium-high heat, then add the oil and bacon. Cook for 3 to 5 minutes, or until the bacon is crispy. Transfer to a paper towel–lined plate and set aside.

3 Add the asparagus, then the reserved pasta water. Cook for 2 minutes, or until the spears are tender when pierced with a fork.

4 Add the cooked pasta, bacon, Parmesan, lemon juice, and salt to the asparagus. Stir gently to combine.

5 Serve immediately.

Tip *If your kids don't like whole wheat pasta, use the Work-Your-Way-Up Strategy (see page 56).*

Zucchini

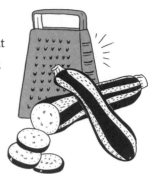

Midway into our 52 New Foods Challenge, I started to experiment with more challenging vegetables like spinach and zucchini. I'm not sure what lured me down this path, but I decided to blend spinach into pancakes. Bad idea. Total fail. Partly because the pancakes tasted awful, but more because my kids didn't want to eat something that they knew was not naturally green.

"Why are the pancakes bright green? Is it food coloring?" inquired Catherine.

Good question! I thought (kicking myself under the table). We had spent months working on knowing what was in our food. Of course they should test and wonder! Announcing it was spinach blended into their pancakes did nothing to help my case. Cardinal rule: No sneaking!

Which brings me to zucchini. Sautéed, baked, or grilled, we tried it countless ways, but Catherine didn't like the texture of zucchini. "Maybe shredded into a muffin?" was my next strategy. But the bits of zuke nestled in her muffin weren't appealing, either. So, together (operative word), we decided to puree it and blend it into our muffins. Full disclosure. "You're eating zucchini! See . . . here it is . . . in the blender . . . in the mixing bowl!"

Success.

As for other ways to enjoy zucchini, we'll keep trying! Next summer we plan to grow it. Maybe we'll have a cauliflower experience—if Catherine grows it, she'll be more likely to enjoy it.

Make It a Game: 15
Eat Your Colors: Green

> ### Invite Exploration
>
> "Do you think zucchini is a vegetable or a fruit? What gives you that idea?"
>
> "What differences do you notice between vegetables and fruits? Is there a way that you can always tell a fruit from a vegetable?"

Zucchini Muffins

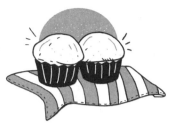

I'm a sucker for a warm basket of fresh-baked muffins. They are fun to make and even more fun to enjoy cuddled up with your kiddos on a Saturday morning.

PREP TIME: 10 minutes
COOK TIME: about 20 minutes
Makes 24 muffins

INGREDIENTS:

2 medium zucchini, trimmed

2 cups whole wheat all-purpose flour

3 teaspoons ground cinnamon

1½ teaspoons baking soda

¾ teaspoon baking powder

1 teaspoon kosher salt

3 large eggs

½ cup light brown sugar

½ cup grapeseed oil

½ cup applesauce

¼ cup flax meal

2 teaspoons pure vanilla extract

Cook Together

Beginners: Shred or puree the zucchini. Measure, mix, and pour.

DIRECTIONS:

1 Preheat the oven to 350°F. Line a standard muffin tin with baking cups. If using silicone cups, my personal preference, spray lightly with olive oil.

2 Chop the zucchini into large pieces, place them in a food processor, and process for 2 minutes, or until the mixture is a consistent, light green color with no large chunks remaining. Set aside. (This step can be done a day ahead and the puree can be stored in the refrigerator.)

3 In a medium bowl, whisk together the flour, cinnamon, baking soda, baking powder, and salt.

4 In the bowl of a stand mixer fitted with the whisk attachment, combine the eggs, sugar, oil, applesauce, flax meal, vanilla, and zucchini puree and beat on medium speed until blended.

5 In small batches, add the flour mixture to the zucchini mixture. Mix on low speed to combine.

6 Divide the batter evenly among the muffin cups, filling each cup about three-quarters full. Bake for 20 to 25 minutes, or until the tops are golden brown and spring back when touched lightly.

Recipe inspired by my friend and fellow mom Kelsey Banfield, author of The Naptime Chef.

Keep Trying Don't assume that your kids won't like shredded zucchini in their muffins. Let them do the preparation and then try it both ways. Just don't hide it!

Easy Cheesy Zucchini

This simple sauté is another easy way to try zucchini. It's quick, which makes it perfect for adding more color to your table on a weeknight.

PREP TIME: 5 minutes

COOK TIME: 5 minutes

Serves 4

INGREDIENTS:

1 tablespoon extra-virgin olive oil

2 medium zucchini, cut into ¼-inch pieces

Kosher salt

Grated Parmesan cheese, for serving

DIRECTIONS:

1 Heat a frying pan over medium-high heat. Add the oil and zucchini and sauté for 3 to 5 minutes, or until the edges brown.

2 Season with the salt and Parmesan before serving.

Grow It When spring temperatures turn warm, and you're well past the risk of frost, it's time to plant zucchini. Enjoy eating both the blossoms and the fruit.

Grilled Zucchini

During the summer, we love to make our meals on the grill and enjoy the pleasure of eating outside. Zucchini is one of our top picks.

PREP TIME: 5 minutes

COOK TIME: 7 to 9 minutes

Serves 4

INGREDIENTS:

2 medium zucchini, halved lengthwise into the shape of boats

1 tablespoon extra-virgin olive oil

1 tablespoon fresh lemon juice (from ½ lemon)

Kosher salt

DIRECTIONS:

1 Preheat a grill to medium heat.

2 Paint each slice of zucchini with the oil. This is a fun job for the kids.

3 Grill the zucchini, cut-side down, for 5 to 7 minutes, or until grill marks appear. Turn and grill for 2 minutes more, until the zucchini is tender.

4 Season with the lemon juice and a sprinkle of salt.

5 Serve immediately.

Zucchini Ribbons

A variation on Rainbow Ribbons (page 85), this easy recipe is a great way to try raw zucchini. It's another way to experiment with taste and texture and a quick way to add color to your table—no cooking required!

PREP TIME: 10 minutes

COOK TIME: 0 minutes

Serves 4

INGREDIENTS:

2 medium zucchini

1 tablespoon extra-virgin olive oil

1 tablespoon fresh lemon juice (from ½ lemon)

¼ teaspoon kosher salt

Grated Parmesan cheese

DIRECTIONS:

1 Using a vegetable peeler, shave the zucchini into long, thin ribbons.

2 In a medium bowl, combine the zucchini ribbons with the oil, lemon juice, and salt. Cover and place in the refrigerator for 15 minutes to let the flavors meld.

3 Sprinkle with grated Parmesan before serving.

Cook Together When peeling the zucchini, remind kids to shave *away* from themselves.

Keep Trying Invite your kids to try zucchini raw versus sautéed or grilled. Let them decide which way they prefer.

Eggplant

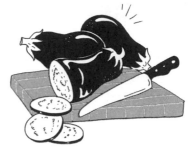

"The trick to eggplant Parmesan? Don't use eggplant." Standing in my friend Cheri's kitchen, chatting about the best way to make eggplant Parmesan, this is the quip that I hear from her witty, and often quiet, husband. It pretty much sums up the reaction I got from most of my friends when I announced we were experimenting with eggplant. But for each vehement opponent, there was a passionate follower, like my mom, who loves eggplant. You either love it or hate it. I was treading in rocky waters.

Eggplant Parmesan seemed like our best shot if we were going to have any success with eggplant. I knew it would be fun to cook together because there was a great deal of dipping, flipping, and sprinkling. The combination of bread crumbs and melted cheese would surely entice even the most reluctant eggplant eater (myself included).

So we called in the big guns and placed a few calls to the resident Italian grandmas (aka our mothers). The secret: no baking! "Healthier" versions of this recipe call for baking the breaded eggplant, but our family experts shot down that idea in favor of taste. Which is a really important point! It's generally healthier to bake rather than fry anything, eggplant included. But this is a case where you bend the rules, because serving mushy eggplant that doesn't taste good won't help your case. It's better to just let it simmer in the pan with some good olive oil and enjoy it. Or choose to make something else. As for Catherine and James, they were surprised how much they loved the crispy rounds fresh off the pan (no tomato sauce required). As for me, I finally discovered a reason to enjoy eggplant.

Make It a Game: 15 points
Eat Your Colors: Blue/Purple

Invite Exploration

"I wonder what would make our eggplant extra crispy?"

Eggplant Parmesan

A classic Italian eggplant parmigiana courtesy of the Italian grandmas who know their stuff when it comes to family-style cooking. The first time I tried this recipe, I left the eggplant in the pan a little too long, but it worked to my advantage. The extra crispiness of the eggplant was what did the trick for my kids (and me)—no mushiness at all!

PREP TIME: 30 minutes

WAIT TIME: 45 minutes

COOK TIME: 20 minutes

Serves 8

INGREDIENTS:

2 medium eggplants

1 tablespoon kosher salt

¾ cup grated Parmesan cheese

¾ cup whole wheat bread crumbs

3 large eggs

1 cup whole wheat flour

6 tablespoons extra-virgin olive oil

6 cups Gram's Homemade Tomato Sauce (page 253)

1½ cups shredded mozzarella cheese

A few sprigs of fresh basil

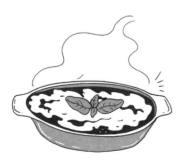

DIRECTIONS:

1 Cut the eggplant into slices no more than ¼ inch thick.

2 Place a wire rack inside a rimmed baking sheet. Line the rack with paper towels.

3 In a large bowl, toss the eggplant together with the salt. Transfer the salted eggplant to the lined wire rack. Let stand 30 to 45 minutes, or until the eggplant releases most

---

Cook Together

Beginners: Run the Eggplant Parmesan assembly line.

Experts: Slice. Sauté.

Tip: Set the bowls of ingredients up like an assembly line and let your kids have fun!

The Secret to Perfect Eggplant Parmesan

The secret to Eggplant Parmesan is to fry it! Take these tips from our Italian moms:

1. Slice it thin. No more than ¼ inch thick.
2. Salt it. Salting draws out the excess moisture.
3. Flour first. Then egg. Then the bread crumb and Parmesan mixture.
4. No baking. Lightly frying in olive oil is the only way to get it crispy.
5. Good sauce. Enough said.

of its liquid. Cover with more paper towels and press firmly to remove the remaining liquid. Wipe off any excess salt.

4 Preheat the oven to 375°F.

5 In a large bowl, mix together the cheese and bread crumbs. In a separate bowl, whisk the eggs. Place the flour in a third bowl. Dip each eggplant slice in flour, then in the egg, then in the bread crumb mixture. Set the breaded slices on the wire rack.

6 Heat a large sauté pan over medium heat, then add the oil and one-third of the breaded eggplant slices. Cook for 3 minutes, or until the bottom turns golden brown and crispy. Flip and cook the second side for 2 minutes more, or until crispy. Repeat, refreshing the oil between batches. Drain the eggplant slices on the wire rack.

7 Spread a layer of tomato sauce on the bottom of a 9 x 13-inch pan. Next, add a layer of eggplant, sprinkle with mozzarella, and add a few sprigs of basil. Repeat.

8 Bake for 20 minutes, or until the sauce is bubbling.

9 Let stand for 5 minutes before serving.

Tip *It is preferable to use homemade tomato sauce, my gram's being my personal favorite, but if not, choose one from a jar with all-natural ingredients you can identify.*

Grilled Eggplant with Minty Yogurt Dip

Like zucchini, eggplant is another great vegetable for the grill. Pair it with a simple, delicious yogurt dip to encourage tasters.

PREP TIME: 5 minutes

COOK TIME: 10 minutes

Serves 4

INGREDIENTS:

1 large eggplant

2 tablespoons extra-virgin olive oil

1 clove garlic, finely chopped

½ cup nonfat plain yogurt

1 tablespoon coarsely chopped fresh mint

1 tablespoon fresh lemon juice (from ½ lemon)

Kosher salt

DIRECTIONS:

1 Slice the eggplant into ¾-inch-thick rounds.

2 In a small bowl, combine the oil and garlic. Using a pastry brush, paint both sides of the eggplant rounds with the garlic mixture.

3 In a small bowl, combine the yogurt, mint, and lemon juice. Set aside.

4 Grill the eggplant slices over medium-high heat for 4 to 5 minutes, then flip and cook for 4 to 5 minutes more, or until grill marks appear. Season with kosher salt to taste.

5 Serve immediately, with the mint-yogurt dipping sauce on the side.

Japanese Eggplant Stir-Fry

My son, James, loves this savory stir-fry. It's delicious alongside Clay-Pot Chicken with Bok Choy (page 130) or Tasty Beef Skewers (page 284).

PREP TIME: 5 minutes

COOK TIME: 8 minutes

Serves 4

INGREDIENTS:

2 small Japanese eggplants

¼ cup Chicken Broth
(page 99)

2 tablespoons tamari or soy
sauce

1 tablespoon grapeseed oil

1 teaspoon finely chopped
garlic

1 teaspoon finely chopped
peeled fresh ginger

Sesame seeds, for sprinkling

DIRECTIONS:

1 Slice the eggplants into ½-inch chunks.

2 In a small bowl, whisk together the broth and tamari.

3 Heat a large wok over medium-high heat, then add the oil, garlic, and ginger and sauté for 30 seconds, or until fragrant. Add the eggplant and cook for 3 to 5 minutes more, until browned.

4 Stir in the broth mixture, reduce the heat to low, and simmer for 3 minutes, or until the sauce thickens and the eggplant softens. Add sesame seed sprinkles before serving.

Keep Trying Focus on the fun of making these recipes together—there's learning even if they don't like it.

Green Beans

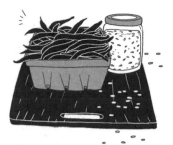

In the early days of our 52 New Foods Challenge, eating our colors gave our plates a boost, but I found that we had about five go-to favorites that kept appearing on the menu. Green beans were one of them. I was certainly not complaining that we had moved beyond pasta and peas, a feat in and of itself, but I was longing for a little variety! I didn't want to mess with a good thing, so instead I slowly started to experiment with simple new ways to enjoy our old favorites.

"How about adding a few sprinkles to those green beans?" I inquired at the table. Okay, "sprinkles" was maybe a bit of an oversell, but I got their attention.

"Let me!" shouted James. He rarely had a chance to beat his sister to the punch, so whenever there was an opening he jumped to the occasion. I handed him the jar of sesame seeds and let him go to town. More "sprinkles" ended up on the table than in the bowl, but I thoroughly enjoyed his enthusiasm—James' defining characteristic.

It was wonderful how that simple little change turned something old into something refreshingly new. The next night, we added a touch of sesame oil and rice vinegar to spice it up—but just a little so that we wouldn't lose the appeal of one of our keystone veggies. Adding sprinkles—sesame seeds, sunflower seeds, flaxseeds, or sliced almonds—is an easy way to brighten your (boring) regulars. It's a small change, but an important part of getting your kids used to the idea of trying old favorites in new ways.

Make It a Game: 10 points
Eat Your Colors: Green, Yellow/Orange, Purple

Invite Exploration

"What other foods would make great sprinkles on our veggies?"

Sesame Green Bean Salad

A simple sesame green bean salad adds a new twist to an old favorite and makes supper super fun! The subtle, nutty flavor of sesame seeds is easy to enjoy and added an Asian twist to one of our weeknight regulars: green beans. This recipe makes a great side for our Clay-Pot Chicken with Bok Choy (page 130) or Ginger-Soy Glazed Cod (page 287).

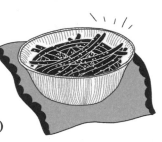

PREP TIME: 5 minutes

COOK TIME: 10 minutes

Serves 4

INGREDIENTS:

1 pound green beans, trimmed

1 tablespoon extra-virgin olive oil

1 teaspoon sesame seeds

DIRECTIONS:

1 In a medium saucepan, bring 2 inches of water to a boil. Place the green beans in a steamer insert and set them over the boiling water. Cook the beans for 5 to 7 minutes, or until they are bright green and tender when pierced with a fork. Steam them a little less if you prefer your beans on the crunchy side. Drain the beans and give them a bath in a large bowl of ice water to bring back their color. Drain again and place in a large bowl.

2 In a medium bowl, mix together the oil and green beans. Let your kids add the sprinkles (aka sesame seeds). Toss gently to coat.

Tip *Add ½ teaspoon sesame oil if you'd like to take the flavor up a notch.*

Cook Together

Beginners: Snap ends off the beans. Give the beans a bath. Mix the dressing. Add the sprinkles!

Experts: Cook the beans.

Skinny Beans and Almonds

This recipe is made with French beans. They are commonly called haricots verts, but my kids call them "skinny beans."

PREP TIME: 10 minutes

COOK TIME: 7 minutes

Serves 4

INGREDIENTS:

¼ cup sliced almonds

1 pound French beans (haricots verts), trimmed

1 tablespoon extra-virgin olive oil

1 small shallot, finely chopped

Kosher salt

DIRECTIONS:

1 In a small frying pan, toast the almonds over medium-high heat for 3 minutes, or until they are golden brown. Shake the pan to make sure they don't burn.

2 In a medium saucepan, bring 2 inches of water to a boil. Place the beans in a steamer insert and set it in the pan. Cook the beans for 2 to 3 minutes, or until they are bright green and tender when pierced with a fork. (These beans cook faster than regular green beans.) Drain the beans, then give them a bath in ice water. Drain again and set aside.

3 Heat the now-empty pot over medium heat. Add the oil and shallots and sauté for 2 to 3 minutes, or until lightly browned and crispy on the edges.

4 Add the beans, toasted almonds, and salt to the shallots. Toss to combine in the pan.

5 Transfer to a large bowl and serve immediately.

Grow It Beans make a great addition to your kitchen garden. Wait until the risk of frost has passed before you get started. Provide a trellis so they have room to climb. Plant your colors—green, yellow, and purple.

Easy Oven Green Beans

Another easy way to prepare green beans is to bake them in an aluminum foil pocket. My kids love wrapping the beans up like a present! This also works on the grill. Just be careful when you open the package—the hot steam can easily burn little fingers.

PREP TIME: 10 minutes

COOK TIME: 20 minutes

Serves 4

INGREDIENTS:

1 pound green beans, trimmed

1 tablespoon extra-virgin olive oil

3 large cloves garlic

¼ teaspoon kosher salt

1 tablespoon sesame seeds

DIRECTIONS:

1 Preheat the oven to 400°F.

2 Place the beans in the center of a large piece of aluminum foil. Add the oil, garlic, salt, and 1 tablespoon water. Fold the foil over the beans and seal to make a pocket. Shake gently to combine the ingredients in the pouch.

3 Bake for 10 minutes. Turn the pouch and bake for 10 minutes more.

4 Remove the pouch from the oven and open carefully. You'll know the beans are done when they are tender when pierced with a fork.

5 Transfer the beans to a serving dish. Add the sesame seeds and toss gently to combine.

6 Serve immediately.

Keep Trying Add a few slices of fennel to the beans before cooking for an easy variation.

Portobello Mushrooms

Mushrooms (aka "mum mums") have always been a favorite food for Catherine—the single reliable "white" vegetable on the color wheel. It was her love of button mushrooms that led us to portobellos. Big and beefy like a sea captain, those hulking caps show up at the farmers' market and demand attention—the supersize version of mushrooms. Interest piqued, I started cooking up a plan.

At dinner one night, as the button mushrooms were being passed around the table, Catherine commented, "I love mum mums!" The ball bounced to me.

"Yes, and," I replied, "you might want to try these grilled portobellos that Daddy made. Their flavor is similar to the mushrooms you're eating. They are from the same family." The connection was close enough—both in smell and appearance—that Catherine was willing to give them a try. And the results were encouraging.

"What do you think? Do you like them?" I inquired hesitantly.

"Yes, and," Catherine replied with a clever smile, "I'd like a second serving."

The "Yes, and" strategy worked for Catherine and portobellos, and became a tactic that I continued to rely on throughout our 52 New Foods Challenge. Asian pears are like apples and pears mixed together. Rainbow carrots taste like regular carrots, but are more colorful. Fennel is like celery, but with a zing. Whenever you can, try to make these connections for your kids, giving them the stepping-stones they need to continue on the path to a more colorful (and varied) diet.

Make It a Game: 10 points
Eat Your Colors: White/Brown

Invite Exploration

"I wonder why you can eat some mushrooms but not others. How can we tell the difference?"

Grilled Portobello Mushrooms

Grilling is my favorite way to enjoy portobello mushrooms. Who needs a burger when these show up? The favorite part of this recipe for my kids was scooping out the gills of the mushroom. Work over a compost bin or a rimmed baking sheet to minimize the mess.

PREP TIME: 10 minutes

COOK TIME: 5 to 7 minutes

Serves 4

INGREDIENTS:

4 large portobello mushrooms

2 tablespoons extra-virgin olive oil

Kosher salt

Cook Together

Beginners: Scoop out the gills. Paint the caps with olive oil.

Experts: Grill and slice the mushrooms.

DIRECTIONS:

1 Preheat the grill to medium-high.

2 Remove the stems from the mushrooms. Using a spoon, scoop out the gills from the underside of the mushrooms and discard them.

3 Place the mushrooms stem-side down on a rimmed baking sheet. Using a pastry brush, paint the tops of the caps with the oil.

4 Grill the mushrooms, cap-side down, for 3 to 4 minutes, or until grill marks appear. Flip and cook the second side for 2 to 3 minutes more.

5 Let the mushrooms cool slightly, then cut them into ¼-inch slices. Season with kosher salt and serve warm.

Tip *Wash then wipe. The best way to remove dirt from a mushroom is to run it under cool water then wipe it gently with a paper towel.*

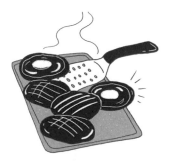

Roasted Portobellos

If you're not able to fire up the grill, roasting portobellos in the oven is another easy way to prepare this burly white vegetable.

PREP TIME: 10 minutes

COOK TIME: 8 to 10 minutes

Serves 4

INGREDIENTS:

4 large portobello mushrooms

4 tablespoons extra-virgin olive oil

Kosher salt

Garlic powder

DIRECTIONS:

1 Preheat the oven to 500°F. Line a rimmed baking sheet with foil.

2 Remove the stems from the mushrooms. Using a spoon, scoop out and discard the gills. Wipe the tops clean with a damp paper towel.

3 Place the mushrooms stem-side down on the baking sheet. Drizzle 1 tablespoon of oil on each cap. Rub in the oil with your fingers to coat thoroughly.

4 Roast for 5 minutes, then flip the caps and cook for 3 to 5 minutes more, or until the mushrooms are charred and tender.

5 Let the mushrooms cool slightly before slicing them into ¼-inch sections. Season with kosher salt and garlic powder before serving.

Buy in Season There are so many wonderful (and unusual) varieties of mushrooms. Head to the farmers' market and see how many different kinds you can find. They are available year-round.

Portobello Mushroom Quesadillas

Need another easy way to feature Roasted Portobellos (page 197) on your table? Make quesadillas! Pair with Black Bean Soup (page 174) for a quick and healthy dinner.

PREP TIME: 10 minutes

COOK TIME: 5 minutes

Serves 4

INGREDIENTS:

4 (8-inch) whole wheat flour tortillas

2 cups grated cheddar cheese

1 recipe Roasted Portobellos (page 197)

DIRECTIONS:

1 In a large sauté pan, warm each tortilla over medium heat for 1 to 2 minutes, or until small bubbles appear.

2 Flip the tortilla, reduce the heat to low, then add ½ cup of the cheese. Sprinkle the cheese evenly over the tortilla, but don't go all the way to the edges. Layer 5 to 6 slices of portobello on one half of the tortilla. Using a spatula, fold the tortilla in half and press down gently. Cook for 1 to 2 minutes, or until the bottom is golden brown and the cheese has melted.

3 Slide the cooked tortilla onto a wooden cutting board.

4 Repeat with the remaining tortillas and filling ingredients.

5 Let the quesadillas cool slightly, then slice into quarters and serve.

Tip For more color, add sliced avocado, apples, or salsa along with your mushrooms.

Peas

With all of my complaining about pasta and peas, you would have good reason to wonder why I would include peas in this book. Let me set the record straight—I don't have it out for peas. But in those early days, I needed a break. Once we crossed the wasteland of white pasta and entered a more colorful place, I was willing to see the merits of peas.

Shell peas are one of the most fun spring vegetables for kids. Peeling back the curly string, then opening the pod to reveal the tiny green pearls snuggled inside is the vegetable equivalent to opening a candy wrapper. The tender taste of freshly shelled peas, whether picked from your garden gate or your local farmers' market, is refreshing beyond compare. My preference is for garden-fresh peas but frozen can be good, too. Here's why: First, frozen peas are easy—to find (most every grocery store has them), to keep (an informal poll found frozen peas in most households with young children), and to cook (just toss them into sauces, pasta dishes, or salads for an extra splash of color). Second, frozen vegetables, like peas, in some cases can be more nutritious than fresh. When peas are picked at their peak and frozen at the site, it locks in the nutrients. Often, fresh grocery store peas have traveled from a faraway land, shedding some of their nutritional value and flavor along the way (which explains that unwelcome gritty taste). If you have the choice, freshly picked peas from your garden or local farmers' market are best, but frozen can be good, too (just maybe not as flavorful). Let the peas that have landed in the produce aisle of your grocery store be your third choice—and definitely skip the can when you can, to avoid the BPA.

Make It a Game: 10 points
Eat Your Colors: Green

Invite Exploration

"How would you describe the flavor of fresh peas eaten straight from the pod?"

Fresh Buttered Peas

This simple dish is arguably one of the best ways to enjoy fresh English peas. The joy of this recipe (if you can call it that) is the shelling—a favorite activity for my kids that will keep them occupied for a solid twenty minutes. One for you, one for the bowl. Two for you, none for the bowl. When peas are in season, it's a great opportunity to compare the taste of fresh versus frozen, side by side.

PREP TIME: 20 minutes

COOK TIME: 5 minutes

Serves 4

INGREDIENTS:

2 pounds fresh English peas
(about 2 cups shelled)

1 tablespoon unsalted butter

¼ teaspoon kosher salt

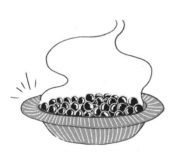

DIRECTIONS:

1 Set your kids up at a table and let them shell the peas.

2 Fill a medium saucepan with water and bring to a boil. Add the peas and cook for 2 to 3 minutes, or until the peas are bright green. Drain and set aside.

3 In the now empty saucepan, melt the butter over low heat. When the butter begins to bubble, but before it starts to turn brown, add the peas and stir gently to coat thoroughly. Season with salt and serve immediately.

Tip *If it's growing in your garden, add 1 tablespoon coarsely chopped fresh mint.*

Tip *To reveal the treasure inside an English pea, snap off the end of the shell and gently pull away from the pod to remove the string. Work over a rimmed baking sheet so that those round gems don't roll off the table.*

> ### Cook Together
>
> **Beginners:** Shell the peas. Heat the butter. Season the peas.

Pea Shooters

The texture of pea soup can be challenging for some (including me and my kids). To avoid overwhelming anyone, serve it in small cups like an eggcup or a demitasse cup to encourage tasters. Add an extra splash of chicken broth if you prefer a lighter texture.

PREP TIME: 10 minutes

COOK TIME: 5 minutes

Serves 4

INGREDIENTS:

2 tablespoons unsalted butter

½ cup finely chopped white onions

2 cups Chicken Broth (page 99)

2½ cups freshly shelled or frozen peas

Kosher salt

Croutons, for garnish

DIRECTIONS:

1 In a large saucepan, melt the butter over medium heat. Add the onions and cook for 2 to 3 minutes, or until translucent and softened.

2 Add the broth to the onions and bring to a boil. Add the peas and cook for 2 to 3 minutes more, or until the peas are bright green.

3 Remove the saucepan from the heat and let the soup cool slightly. Working in small batches, carefully transfer the soup to a blender and puree. (Be careful when blending hot liquids.)

4 Return the soup to the saucepan and warm it over medium-low heat.

5 Season with kosher salt to taste. Garnish with croutons.

Tip *If it's growing in your garden, add a few coarsely chopped fresh mint leaves.*

Cook Together

It's helpful to wrap a kitchen towel around the lid of the blender to protect kids from any hot liquid that might escape as you blend.

Keep Trying
For an even smoother texture, run the soup through a sieve.

Grow It

Tips for Growing Perfect Peas

Step 1: Start Early. If you're starting from seeds, plant your peas as early as March or even February in some areas (plant as early as you can work in the soil).[2] According to expert gardeners, pea plants are hardy enough to endure the cold. Place them in a sunny spot, near a trellis or fence—like a toddler, they like to climb.

Step 2: Pick Often. The trick to getting your pea plant to deliver a big harvest is to pick them—frequently. This shouldn't be a problem. In our house, the bigger challenge was not picking the peas so that we could grow a batch big enough to make something! In late spring or early summer, it's easy to augment your recipes with fresh peas from the farmers' market if your garden doesn't deliver enough.

Blueberries

Blueberries have always been a favorite food for my family. Highly transportable in little snack boxes and the perfect size for small fingers, blueberries were a frequent fruit when both Catherine and James were toddlers. Even now, when buckets of berries arrive at the market, we stock up—maximizing their volume on our seasonal menu and stowing away a few big bags in the freezer to save for winter days when we need a good berry blast to scare away colds and other creaky winter ailments. Don't be fooled by their diminutive size—blueberries are packed with powerful anthocyanins, which is where they get their color.[3] Free radicals, meet Mighty Mouse.

It turns out blueberries had another benefit. They were a great way to get my kids to try new foods. Like mandarin oranges, blueberries were a Gateway Food for us (see page 14). Serving them as part of a rainbow salad bar, I was able to get my kids to try radicchio, jícama, and mango. Blueberries formed the foundation, so they were willing to try a little of something new along with them.

Use blueberries as a building block. Start by pairing them with lime juice and tossing in a few juicy chunks of fresh mango—more or less depending on how adventurous your kids are feeling. Ready to take it up a notch? Add jícama, red onion, and tomatillos to make a salsa. If the more subtle approach suits your style, blend blueberries into a smoothie along with a new food like flaxseeds. Those little blue gems pack a big benefit when it comes to adding healthy color to your family table.

Make It a Game: 5 points
Eat Your Colors: Blue/Purple

Invite Exploration

"Which new foods can we try with blueberries? Can you come up with an unusual combination?"

Blueberry-Mango Salad

This simple salad serves as a great vehicle for trying new foods like mango, jícama, radicchio, red onion, and tomatillo. Use blueberries as the base, and let your kids have fun mixing it up.

PREP TIME: 5 minutes

WAIT TIME: 30 to 60 minutes

Serves 4

INGREDIENTS:

1 pint fresh blueberries
(about 2 cups)

1 large Manila mango, peeled
and diced

1 tablespoon fresh lime juice
(from 1 lime)

1 tablespoon fresh cilantro
leaves (optional)

DIRECTIONS:

1 In a large bowl, gently combine the blueberries, mango, lime juice, and cilantro leaves (if using).

2 Chill for 30 to 60 minutes, to let the flavors meld.

3 Use your Blueberry-Mango Salad as a base. Serve with other new foods like jícama (sliced thin and tossed with lemon or lime), radicchio (shaved fine), red onions (chopped fine), or tomatillos (roasted or raw) and invite your kids to make a new mix to try. Encourage each person to make one for themselves and two to share.

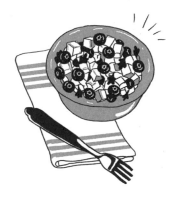

Cook Together

Beginners: Squeeze the juice. Assemble the salads.

Experts: Dice the fruit and vegetables.

Blueberry Blast Smoothie

This refreshing smoothie is a blast of healthy goodness. Use it as a base for trying new foods, like flax- or chia seeds. In the spring, when blueberries are in season, be sure to freeze a big bag of them, along with fresh mint, so that you can enjoy this smoothie any time of year.

PREP TIME: 5 minutes

COOK TIME: 0 minutes

Serves 4

INGREDIENTS:

1 cup blueberries (fresh or frozen)

1 banana, peeled

½ cup nonfat plain yogurt

½ cup freshly squeezed orange juice

4 or 5 ice cubes

1 tablespoon fresh lemon juice (from ½ lemon)

1 tablespoon coarsely chopped fresh mint leaves, plus whole leaves for garnish

DIRECTIONS:

1 In a blender, combine the blueberries, banana, yogurt, orange juice, ice cubes, lemon juice, and mint leaves. Blend until smooth, about 2 minutes.

2 Pour into glasses, garnish with mint leaves, and serve immediately.

Tip To save garden-fresh mint for your smoothies, wash it thoroughly, chop it, place it in an ice cube tray, fill with water, and freeze. Pop the cubes in your blender for a refreshing boost of mint in smoothies all year long.

Buy in Season To keep seasonal berries fresh longer, wait to wash them until you're ready to eat. Remember to freeze a few pints for use in the winter.

Cinnamon-Blueberry Awesome Sauce

This sauce is delicious drizzled over pancakes, crepes, or French toast. It's also tasty swirled into yogurt parfaits. Pair it with fruits like kiwi, raspberries, and peaches. The combination will make your kids forget that they ever liked flavored yogurts.

PREP TIME: 5 minutes

COOK TIME: 5 minutes

Serves 4

INGREDIENTS:

1 cup blueberries

1 tablespoon honey

1 tablespoon fresh lemon juice
(from ½ lemon)

¼ teaspoon ground cinnamon

DIRECTIONS:

1 In a small saucepan over medium heat, combine the blueberries, honey, lemon juice, cinnamon, and 2 tablespoons water. Bring to a boil, then reduce the heat to maintain a simmer and cook for 5 minutes, or until the mixture resembles syrup.

2 Serve warm or cold.

Strawberries

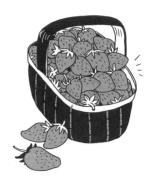

Eyes squinting, I follow the cloud that rises as Catherine and James tear down the dusty trail. The sweltering heat does nothing to slow their stride. Like journalists on the hunt for a hot tip, they work together to scout the best location. Hitting the jackpot, they stay crouched close to the bushes, carefully picking their treasure. It's an activity that captures their attention for hours: berry picking.

There is something thrilling about venturing into a wide-open farm field, little pails in hand, to find and pick your own bounty of juicy fruit. Maybe it's the pleasure of eating fruit straight from the vine, or the excitement of standing face-to-face with thousands of sweet buds lining the carefully laid rows of strawberry bushes. Whatever the reason, berry picking provides a jam-packed morning for the whole family. It's an activity I'd highly recommend when strawberries are in season.

Start by finding a local, pick-your-own farm (localharvest.org is a great resource for finding farms near you). Seek out farms that are certified organic. When grown conventionally, strawberries are considered part of the Dirty Dozen, which means they can be laden with pesticides (see page 42). Bring two pails: one for ripe fruit, the other for just-past-ripe fruit. Farmers will often give you the just-past-ripe fruit for free, especially if you help them pick it, and it's perfect for making jam or fruit leather. Save a portion of your bounty for freezing. You'll appreciate those sweet berries in smoothies when the winter blues hit.

Make It a Game: 5 points
Eat Your Colors: Red

> ### Invite Exploration
>
> "I wonder how you can tell which plants will bear the most fruit?"
>
> "Can you think of an easy way to hull a strawberry?"

Healthy Strawberry Fool

This easy recipe is a simple spin on an old-fashioned treat: strawberry fool. We swapped out the whipped cream for yogurt and added a touch of honey to sweeten the mix. It's also a great way to wean your kids off flavored yogurt, which is generally made with as much sugar as ice cream and is deceptively unhealthy. To break the habit, encourage your kids to make their own blend with simple, wholesome ingredients.

PREP TIME: 5 minutes

COOK TIME: 0 minutes

Serves 4

INGREDIENTS:

3 cups strawberries

1½ cups nonfat plain yogurt

2 tablespoons honey

2 tablespoons fresh lemon juice (from 1 lemon)

Fresh mint sprigs, for garnish

Fresh berries, for garnish (optional)

Granola, for serving

DIRECTIONS:

1 Wash, hull, and chop the strawberries into ½-inch pieces.

2 Place the cut fruit in a medium bowl. Using a potato masher, crush the fruit. Allow a few chunks to remain.

3 Add the yogurt, honey, and lemon juice to the strawberries. Fold gently to combine.

4 Serve with a sprig of mint, or a fresh berry on top, and a sprinkle of granola.

Tip To easily hull a strawberry, cut off the top of the berry, then the tip. Using a chopstick, gently poke through the middle of the fruit. Remove the hull with your fingers.

> ### Cook Together
>
> **Beginners:** Hull the strawberries. Mash the fruit. Squeeze the lemon juice. Mix the yogurt.
>
> **Experts:** Cut the fruit.

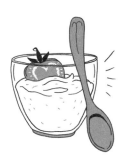

Strawberry Sauce

This is a terrific alternative to syrup for pancakes or crepes. Tasty on yogurt, too! Make it on a Sunday, and use it to dress up breakfasts all week long.

PREP TIME: 10 minutes
COOK TIME: 0 minutes
Makes 1 cup

INGREDIENTS:

½ pint strawberries

1 tablespoon honey

DIRECTIONS:

1 Wash, hull, and roughly chop the strawberries.

2 Place the strawberries, honey, and 1 tablespoon water in a blender. Blend for 2 minutes, or until the mixture is smooth.

3 Store in an airtight container in your refrigerator for up to 1 week.

Grow It

Slugs were a big problem with our strawberry plants. We had much more success with a large container placed in a sunny location. Look for everbearing, or day-neutral, varieties that will bear fruit through the summer into early fall.

Plums

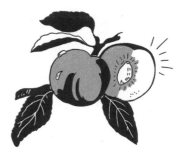

When Catherine was a toddler, a big plum tree graced our backyard. The canopy of that lovely tree provided the perfect shade for picnics, and as late spring turned into early summer, it delivered the best gift of all: fresh plums. Lots of them! Together we would gather them up in paper bags and give them away to friends and neighbors. There were far too many for us to enjoy on our own, and it was much more fun to give them away anyhow. If we weren't fast enough, the squirrels would feast.

A house remodel left our garden in disarray, and unfortunately, our friend the plum tree didn't make it. Every store-bought plum was a faint reminder of our homegrown fruit, but never quite achieved the same wonderful taste and texture.

That all changed at the farmers' market one morning. Strolling up to the stands on one of our weekly trips, we were greeted with crates of plums. Not only the deep purple, deliciously sweet kind that used to fall from our tree, but bright yellow Shiro plums, tangy Santa Rosa beauties, and the sweetly sour Dapple Dandy—a cross between a plum and an apricot that has become a fast favorite in our house. Handpicked from a nearby farm, the fruit was perfectly ripe with a taste far superior to anything found at the grocery store. My kids were fascinated by the range of plum varieties, and had fun comparing notes on flavors, colors, sizes, and shapes. Baskets filled to the brim, we headed home to try all kinds of different plums in all kinds of different ways!

Make It a Game: 5 points
Eat Your Colors: Red, Blue/Purple

Invite Exploration

"How many different varieties of plums can you find? What differences do you notice between the different types?"

Roasted Plums with Pistachios

Baking fruit is one of our favorite ways to make dessert and is another easy way to work in your colors. Warm and juicy with a touch of honey, these roasted plums are an easy treat that is not too sweet—a delicious dessert that takes very little effort.

PREP TIME: 5 minutes

COOK TIME: 20 to 25 minutes

Serves 4

INGREDIENTS:

4 large plums

½ cup honey

1 tablespoon unsalted butter

1 tablespoon fresh lemon juice (from ½ lemon)

2 tablespoons roasted unsalted pistachios

½ cup plain yogurt or vanilla ice cream, for serving

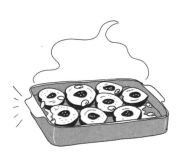

DIRECTIONS:

1 Preheat the oven to 400°F.

2 Slice the plums in half. Remove the pits and discard them. Place the fruit in a medium baking dish.

3 In a small saucepan, warm the honey, butter, and lemon juice over low heat, stirring gently until combined.

4 Drizzle the honey mixture over the fruit. Using a large spoon, turn the fruit in the mixture to coat thoroughly. Arrange the plums cut-side down.

5 Bake for 10 minutes, then turn the plums and bake for 10 to 15 minutes more, or until the fruit is tender but not mushy.

6 While the plums are baking, chop the pistachios. Place the shelled nuts in a sealed plastic bag. On a cutting board, let the kids smash the nuts with a rolling pin until roughly chopped.

7 When cooked, transfer the plums to individual serving bowls, drizzle with syrup from the baking dish, add a spoonful of yogurt or ice cream, and sprinkle with pistachios. Serve immediately.

Cook Together

Beginners: Remove the pits. Squeeze the lemon juice. Smash the nuts.

Experts: Slice the plums. Cook the sauce.

Tip: Use a melon baller to remove the pits. This will be much easier than trying to use a knife, especially for young kids.

Asian Plum Sauce

This tasty, tangy sauce is perfect paired with Easy Roasted Chicken (page 282) or Gigi's Roasted Pork Tenderloin (page 286). Sauces like this one add a boost of color to your table, too!

PREP TIME: 10 minutes

COOK TIME: 18 minutes

Makes 2 cups

INGREDIENTS:

4 large plums

1 clove garlic, finely chopped

1 coin peeled fresh ginger, finely chopped

2 tablespoons rice vinegar

1 tablespoon light brown sugar

DIRECTIONS:

1 Slice the plums in half. Remove the pits and discard them. Cut the fruit into quarters.

2 In a medium saucepan over medium heat, combine the plums, garlic, ginger, rice vinegar, and sugar. Cook for 2 to 3 minutes, then reduce the heat to low and simmer for 15 minutes, stirring occasionally and breaking up the plums, until the fruit breaks down into large chunks and the sauce thickens.

Buy in Season The perfect plum will be plump and will give just a little when gently squeezed. These are best for enjoying right at the stand! Pick a few that are on the firm side and leave them in a paper bag at room temperature for a day or two to ripen.

Keep Trying Try lots of different varieties of plums to reinforce the habit of trying something new. Challenge your kids to find at least three different varieties at the farmers' market. Compare tastes.

Cherries

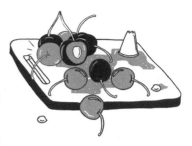

Pop, pop, pop! Like popping corn, cherry trees explode with tiny pink flowers—a telltale sign that warmer weather is ahead. Strolling through our neighborhood in early spring, Catherine noticed a small grove of cherry trees, their delicate branches hanging heavy with ripe, red cherries. "Let's make cherries our new food this week!" she cheered. When cherries come to town for their brief but lovely visit, we are all in!

I love cherries, but with a hint of reservation. Don't get me wrong—I will never turn down a piece of homemade cherry pie. But sitting for hours on end pitting cherries is not my idea of a good time. A pitter may be a convenient gadget when it comes to making anything that requires a big batch of cherries, but in the service of clutter control, it's a kitchen tool that I can live without. And then there are the stains!

However, to try cherries a few different ways, we needed to get rid of those pits en masse—the perfect problem for my kids to solve. The challenge: remove the pits without damaging the fruit. I did a little research to seed some ideas and placed a paring knife, a straw, a bobby pin, and a star-shaped pastry tip on a cutting board and let my kids experiment (outside). Catherine and James dove into their work, slicing and poking and prodding, experimenting to find the optimal cherry pitting method that was equally as fun as it was easy. In the end, the pastry tip won first prize. It's a messy job, to be sure, but one that had my kids captivated for a good thirty minutes and delivered a sweet reward like no other.

Make It a Game: 5 points
Eat Your Colors: Red

Invite Exploration

"How would you pit a cherry without a pitter?"

Simple Cherry Compote

Life's a bowl of cherries—especially when you're enjoying the simple pleasures of homemade cherry compote. This compote is delicious drizzled over homemade vanilla ice cream or swirled into yogurt.

PREP TIME: 30 minutes

COOK TIME: 10 to 12 minutes

Serves 4

INGREDIENTS:

1 pint fresh cherries

1 tablespoon honey

Vanilla ice cream, for serving (optional)

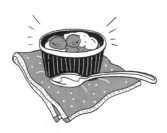

DIRECTIONS:

1 Wash and pit the cherries. This part is messy, but great fun for the kids!

2 Combine the honey and ½ cup water in a small saucepan. Bring to a gentle boil, then reduce the heat to low and simmer, uncovered, until a thin syrup forms, 5 to 7 minutes.

3 Add the cherries. Cook for 5 minutes more, stirring occasionally. (Cook longer for a more jammy texture.)

4 Serve warm, over homemade vanilla ice cream, or let cool completely and add to your favorite yogurt parfait.

Cook Together

Beginners: Pit the cherries.

Experts: Cook the compote.

Tip: It's easy to pit cherries without a pitter—no need for special kitchen gadgets. Instead, we use a simple tool that's already in our pantry: a pastry tip. My kids love this pitting project—but be warned, it can get messy! Be sure to wear clothes that can handle a stain or two.

1. Remove the stems from the cherries.
2. Place the cherry stem-side down on the top of a star-shaped metal pastry tip.
3. Using your fingers to hold the sides of the fruit, press down gently, and presto—out pops the pit!

Cherry Parfaits

Who doesn't love a parfait? Just saying the word makes you feel happy. This recipe is another delicious way to enjoy your Simple Cherry Compote (page 214).

PREP TIME: 5 minutes

COOK TIME: 0 minutes

Serves 4

INGREDIENTS:

½ cup Simple Cherry Compote (page 214)

2 cups nonfat plain yogurt

Pitted fresh cherries, for serving

¼ cup granola, for serving

Honey, for serving

DIRECTIONS:

1   Prepare a batch of Simple Cherry Compote.

2   Line up four small glasses or parfait dishes on the counter. Scoop 2 tablespoons of the compote into the bottom of each cup.

3   Layer ½ cup of yogurt over the compote in each glass. Top the yogurt with a small handful of fresh cherries, a sprinkle of granola, and a drizzle of honey.

Sour Cherry Blasters

These aren't the crazy candies you find at the corner convenience store. We've always called dried cherries Sour Cherry Blasters. They are easy to make at home. This recipe takes some patience—not only pitting the cherries but also waiting while those bright buds transform in your oven. The reward is worth the wait. Enjoy them as a lunchbox snack or baked into oatmeal cookies.

PREP TIME: 30 minutes
COOK TIME: 6 to 8 hours
Serves 4

INGREDIENTS:
1 pound cherries

DIRECTIONS:

1 Preheat the oven to 150°F. Line a rimmed baking sheet with parchment paper.

2 Remove the stems and pits from the cherries and discard them.

3 Place the pitted cherries on the lined baking sheet and let dry in the oven for 6 to 8 hours, or until the fruit is shriveled and turns a deep purplish-red color.

Cook Together

Sweet Bing cherries are likely the easiest to source at your local market, but if you can find the Montmorency variety, they are a wonderfully sour treat.

Buy in Season Cherries pack a punch, made stronger when they are freshly picked! Those little red buds are rich in phytonutrients, and research suggests that powerful antioxidants are at their highest potential when the fruit is freshly picked. Yet another good reason to enjoy cherries when they are in season![4]

Rhubarb

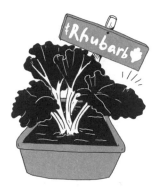

Bubbling around the edges of the crust and dripping over the edge of the pan, it was impossible for little fingers to resist swiping a taste of the sweet blend of tender strawberries, warm honey, and rhubarb. It was my daughter's first encounter with this tough vegetable, and had they met any other way, they might not have become friends.

Rhubarb was one of the many vegetables that Catherine and her classmates had been growing in their school garden. The gigantic leaves of this plant were quite a spectacle—big enough to provide welcome shade for sun-drenched kindergarteners and small animals alike. The same magic that had worked its wonders with Catherine and cauliflower had struck again with rhubarb. Her willingness to try this new food was greatly enhanced by the fact that she had a hand in growing it. Homemade strawberry rhubarb crisp was a well-deserved reward for a hard day's work tending the plants.

Aside from the all-important aspect of adding variety to your menu, rhubarb goes a long way to breaking down stereotypes. I love that it's a veggie you can enjoy as dessert (just like the more predictable carrots, pumpkin, and zucchini). Some argue that dessert is the only way to enjoy rhubarb because of its sour taste. One thing I'm constantly reinforcing—mostly for myself because I have the sweet tooth in our family—is that fruit can be dessert. A sweet ending to a delicious meal doesn't have to be dominated by chocolate. Even better when dessert is a vegetable!

Make It a Game: 15 points
Eat Your Colors: Red

Invite Exploration

"I wonder what makes rhubarb leaves poisonous, but the stalks edible?"

Strawberry-Rhubarb Crisp

This book wouldn't be complete without Catherine's favorite Strawberry-Rhubarb Crisp, an easier version of rhubarb pie. After all, rhubarb's infamous nickname is "pie plant."

PREP TIME: 10 minutes

COOK TIME: 60 minutes

Serves 8

INGREDIENTS:

FOR THE FILLING:

1½ pounds red rhubarb stalks, chopped (about 4 cups)

1½ pounds strawberries, hulled and chopped (about 4 cups)

¼ cup honey

¼ cup maple syrup

2 tablespoons whole wheat all-purpose flour

FOR THE TOPPING:

1¼ cups whole wheat all-purpose flour

1 cup old-fashioned rolled oats

16 tablespoons (2 sticks) unsalted butter, cold, cut into chunks

¼ cup flax meal

½ cup light brown sugar

DIRECTIONS:

1 Preheat the oven to 350°F. Line a rimmed baking sheet with parchment paper.

2 Make the filling: In a large bowl, combine the rhubarb, strawberries, honey, maple syrup, and flour. Set aside.

3 Make the topping: In a separate large bowl, combine the flour, oats, butter, flax meal, and sugar. Using your hands, mix the dough together until it looks like large crumbles.

4 Pour the filling into a large pie plate and cover with the topping. Place the pie plate on the lined baking sheet and bake for 55 to 60 minutes, or until the fruit is bubbling and the topping is golden brown.

5 Serve warm.

Tip *Rhubarb pie can be a bit soupy. To reduce the moisture, try this trick, courtesy of* Cook's Illustrated *(one of my favorite cooking resources): Heat 2 teaspoons grapeseed oil in a saucepan over medium-high heat, then add the rhubarb and cook for 3 to 5 minutes, until it releases most of its liquid but hasn't turned soggy. Let cool before combining with the strawberries. This step takes extra time, so I often skip it and just enjoy the juicy fruit filling, but it can help if you're looking for a firmer texture.*

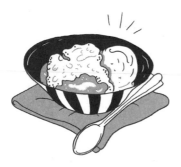

Cook Together

Beginners: Hull the strawberries. Combine the ingredients. Assemble the crisp.

Experts: Cut the rhubarb stalks.

Tip: For younger kids, it's easier to divide the topping mixture into two smaller bowls. Work over a rimmed baking sheet to contain the mess.

Rhubarb Ice Pops

One of our favorite local ice-cream stands makes homemade rhubarb ice cream in the spring. It marks the season. This ice pop recipe is a riff on that signature treat. A little bit tart and a little bit sweet, with a smooth and creamy texture, these pops are so delicious. Any time I make them, they disappear in a flash.

PREP TIME: 5 minutes

COOK TIME: 12 minutes

Makes about 8 ice pops

INGREDIENTS:

2 to 3 rhubarb stalks, cut into ½-inch pieces (about 2 cups chopped)

¼ cup honey

2 tablespoons fresh lemon juice (from 1 lemon)

1 cup nonfat plain yogurt

2 tablespoons maple syrup

DIRECTIONS:

1 In a saucepan, combine the rhubarb, honey, and lemon juice. Simmer over medium-low heat for 10 minutes, or until the rhubarb is soft and the mixture looks like a thick puree. Set aside to cool.

2 In a blender, combine the yogurt, maple syrup, and the cooled rhubarb-honey mixture. Blend until combined, about 2 minutes.

3 Pour the mixture into an ice-pop mold and freeze for about 1 hour. Or use a Zoku pop maker, and your pops will be ready in just a few minutes.

Buy in Season At the market, look for stalks that are sturdy and a vibrant red color.

Grow It Rhubarb is a perennial, which means its spring leaves will pop up year after year with limited assistance on your part. Plant in the early spring, but do not harvest in the first year—rhubarb needs time (and space) to establish itself. This is an occasion when you don't encourage kids to experiment with using the whole plant! You can eat rhubarb stems but not the leaves—they are poisonous.[5]

Sunflower Butter

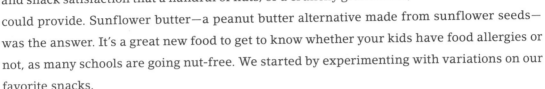

When our school went nut-free, I found myself scrambling for a
lunchbox alternative that could deliver the same energy boost
and snack satisfaction that a handful of nuts, or a crunchy granola bar,
could provide. Sunflower butter—a peanut butter alternative made from sunflower seeds—
was the answer. It's a great new food to get to know whether your kids have food allergies or
not, as many schools are going nut-free. We started by experimenting with variations on our
favorite snacks.

The issue of snacking brings on the same level of debate (and confusion) as how to get
your kids to sleep through the night. So I'll come right out and put my stake in the ground.
Bring on the snacks—but when you do, choose healthy ones. For my kids (and for me) it
works best to offer two healthy snacks a day—one between breakfast and lunch, then one
again between lunch and dinner. A high-protein snack in between meals will stabilize your
body's keel—calming the snack waters enough to avoid major meltdowns. It helps avoid having to negotiate, usually unsuccessfully, with a hungry, weary child.

Sunflower butter is a delicious snack option and can be substituted in most recipes that
call for peanut butter. Although nuts and seeds have higher fat content than protein, which
translates into higher calories, they are considered a healthy choice when eaten in moderation as part of a balanced diet.[6] I try to have tasty snacks, made with this wholesome ingredient, close at hand so that they are just as easy to grab as the less nutritious ones.

Make It a Game: 10 points
Eat Your Colors: Protein

Bitty Bites

The favorite snack food in our house is one that my daughter, Catherine, named Bitty Bites. A no-bake cookie made with sunflower butter, it's great as a lunchbox snack, after-school bite, or post-game energy recharger. Bonus: It's easy and fun for your kids to make. You don't need to be exact with the measurements, which means you can give lots of creative freedom to your kids.

PREP TIME: 5 minutes

WAIT TIME: 15 minutes

Makes about 24 cookies

INGREDIENTS:

1 cup old-fashioned rolled oats (not the quick-cooking kind)

½ cup whole wheat all-purpose flour

½ cup sunflower butter

½ cup honey

¼ cup dark chocolate chips or dried fruit, such as cranberries or raisins

¾ cup shredded unsweetened coconut

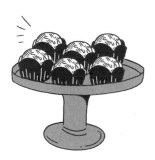

DIRECTIONS:

1 In a food processor, pulse the oats until finely ground, about 2 minutes.

2 Add the flour, sunflower butter, honey, and chocolate chips to the oats. Pulse again until the mixture comes together into a large ball, about 2 minutes more.

3 Using a tablespoon, place a small amount of dough in your hands and roll it into a ball the size of a large marble. Roll each cookie in the shredded coconut. At this point, your kids can shape the cookies however they like. My kids usually leave them as bite-size marbles, or press them in the center with their thumb and add a piece of dried fruit for decoration.

4 Refrigerate the cookies for 15 minutes before serving. Store in an airtight container in the refrigerator for up to 1 week, or freeze for up to 1 month.

Cook Together

Beginners: Combine the ingredients. Roll the cookies.

Tip: An alternative is to combine the dough by hand. After pulsing the oats, add all of the ingredients to a large mixing bowl and use your hands, or a spatula, to combine. This is a fun way to let your kids really get into the mix.

Apple Sandwiches

Ditch the bread and make sunflower butter sandwiches with apple slices instead—a riff on the classic peanut butter sandwich.

PREP TIME: 5 minutes
COOK TIME: 0 minutes
Serves 2

INGREDIENTS:
1 large apple (any variety)
2 tablespoons sunflower butter
1 teaspoon honey

DIRECTIONS:

1 Cutting from top to tip, slice the apple into thin wafers, about ¼ inch thick. Trim out the tough core.

2 On half of the slices, spread the sunflower butter, then drizzle with honey.

3 Top with the remaining slices to create a mini sandwich, and serve.

Ants on a Log

Another variation on a classic, pair sunflower butter with celery and raisins for a quick and satisfying snack.

PREP TIME: 5 minutes
COOK TIME: 0 minutes
Serves 2

INGREDIENTS:
4 stalks celery
¼ cup sunflower butter
Raisins

DIRECTIONS:

1 Slice the celery stalks crosswise into thirds, creating 12 logs.

2 Spread 1 teaspoon of the sunflower butter in the channel of each celery log.

3 Top with raisins (or your favorite dried fruit chopped into small pieces).

Salmon

When Catherine was a toddler, seafood regularly appeared on our weekly menu, and she would happily enjoy it all—from mussels to monkfish. But like the subtle change that occurred when Catherine transformed from a baby-faced toddler into a confident preschooler, her willingness to enjoy fish of any kind changed, seemingly overnight. At our lowest point, Catherine outright refused to sit at the table when fish was served. Fish was right up there with onions—a gnarly dragon seemingly impossible to tame.

But I was determined to stick with it. Fish, and salmon in particular, is an excellent source of omega-3 fatty acids, which are an important component of any person's diet, especially children's. Fish wasn't the only way to get these heart-healthy fats. Supplements are readily available, but in general I lean toward getting our nutrients from the food we eat whenever we can. Fish was one of the best vehicles for omega-3s, so I was reluctant to give up.

We sourced our fish from the fresh market—an easier way to find wild-caught salmon. We cooked together. We talked about how fish helps build a strong body. But more than any one of these factors, it was patience that pulled us through. Salmon just kept showing up. In the end, it was consistent, repeated exposure, over a long period of time, that eventually broke down the barrier. We haven't tamed the dragon, but we've learned that it's not as scary as we once thought. Nowadays, when salmon appears on our family table, Catherine will enjoy it without (too much) fuss.

Make It a Game: 10 points
Eat Your Colors: Protein

Invite Exploration

"I wonder why the color of salmon ranges from light to dark pink? What might be a reason for those differences?"

Sesame-Crusted Salmon

The sesame seed crust makes this salmon recipe sing. Personally, I love how easy this recipe is to make. As for my kids, they love the crunchy sesame seed topping. Win-win.

PREP TIME: 10 minutes
COOK TIME: 12 minutes
Serves 4

INGREDIENTS:

¼ cup sesame seeds

4 salmon fillets (about 1 ½ pounds total)

2 teaspoons grapeseed oil

Cook Together

Beginners: Paint the salmon with grapeseed oil. Add the sesame seed topping.

Experts: Sauté the salmon.

DIRECTIONS:

1 In a large sauté pan, lightly toast the sesame seeds over medium-low heat until golden brown and fragrant, about 2 minutes. Set aside to cool in a medium baking dish.

2 Using a pastry brush, paint the flesh side of the salmon with 1 teaspoon of the oil.

3 Press the salmon fillets, flesh-side down, into the toasted seeds to create the topping.

4 Heat a large frying pan over medium heat. Add the remaining 1 teaspoon oil and the salmon, skin-side down. Cook for 3 to 5 minutes, or until the fillets begin to turn light pink.

5 Using a spatula, flip the fillets and cook for 3 to 5 minutes more, or until the fish is cooked but still pink in the center.

6 Serve immediately.

Tip *When choosing salmon fillets, go for the tail. Those pieces won't have bones, which makes the fish easier for kids to eat.*

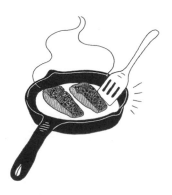

Crispy Salmon Chips

This recipe is tricky but tasty. It's best for a parent to make, kids to enjoy.

PREP TIME: 5 minutes

COOK TIME: 12 to 15 minutes

Serves 4

INGREDIENTS:

1 pound skin-on wild Atlantic salmon

Kosher salt and freshly ground black pepper

DIRECTIONS:

1 Preheat the oven to 400°F. Line a rimmed baking sheet with parchment paper or foil and lightly spray with olive oil to prevent sticking.

2 Place the salmon flesh-side down on a cutting board. With a flat palm, press down on the skin and gently slide a sharp knife between the skin and the flesh to separate. Be careful! Make sure there is as little flesh sticking to the skin as possible. Reserve the flesh for Simple Baked Salmon (page 226).

3 Place the skin, scale-side down, on the prepared baking sheet. Sprinkle with salt and pepper. Bake, turning once, for 12 to 15 minutes, or until crispy.

4 Serve immediately.

Buy in Season Whenever possible, choose fresh, wild salmon over farm-raised. Ask the fishmonger, if it's not clear what you are buying. Let your kids use their keen sense of smell with this food—there should be no fishy smell at all. Choose fish that hasn't been previously frozen, if possible.

Simple Baked Salmon

Sometimes simple is best. This baked salmon is easy to make and is delicious served with Crispy Salmon Chips (page 225). Pair with brown rice and Asparagus with Ginger-Soy Glaze (page 180).

PREP TIME: 5 minutes

COOK TIME: 10 to 15 minutes

Serves 4

INGREDIENTS:

1 pound wild Atlantic salmon, skin removed

1 teaspoon maple syrup

Kosher salt and freshly ground black pepper

Sweet paprika

1 teaspoon grapeseed oil

DIRECTIONS:

1 Preheat the oven to 400°F.

2 Baste the fish with the maple syrup, then season with salt, pepper, and paprika.

3 Heat a large sauté pan over high heat. Add the oil, place the fish in the pan, and sear for 3 to 5 minutes, or until a thin, brown crust forms.

4 Transfer the fish to a rimmed baking sheet and bake for 5 to 10 minutes, or until the fish is light pink in the center.

Keep Trying

For many kids, including Catherine, it can take what seems like an eternity to warm up to fish. Keep trying it lots of different ways and serve it in small portions so as not to overwhelm anyone who is feeling tentative. Head out to the local market to meet a fishmonger as another way to learn about this food.

A Few Things to Know About Fish

Healthy Fats

Omega-3s are the healthy fats found in cold-water fish like salmon. Research suggests that they play an important role in heart health, which is why the American Heart Association recommends eating fish at least twice a week. Many types of seafood contain omega-3s, but salmon has a particularly strong showing in this category, with about one gram of omega-3s per three ounces (about the size of a deck of cards) of fish.[7]

Walk on the Wild Side

When you have the choice, opt for wild salmon over farmed. The concentration of pesticides is lower in these fish.

Check the Guide

When in doubt, check the Seafood Watch website from the Monterey Bay Aquarium (seafoodwatch.org). Their guides will help you determine which fish is safe to eat in your region.

Summer

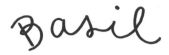# Basil

A distinct and refreshing partner in soups and pasta dishes, basil is one of our favorite garden herbs. Taste aside, I personally love basil because it's easy to grow. It's one of the few crops that I can always rely on, despite my lack of a green thumb. But what if your child picks out those tiny bits of green from anything you prepare like they were ants invading a picnic?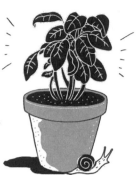

Set up a blind taste test.

Line up three or four small bowls on your table and feature a selection of fresh herbs from your garden or the farmers' market. Basil, mint, parsley, and thyme are all great options—feel free to improvise. Invite your kids into the game with a captivating question like, "Which one smells like cinnamon?" or "Which one tastes like licorice?" Let them pick through the piles, sniffing and sampling. Encourage them to rub the leaves between their fingers to release the fragrant and flavorful oils.

For finicky eaters, this strategy won't banish the fear of flecks of green in their food. But it will get them past that rigid place of absolutely refusing to try it. And in that fun of trying something new, they will discover something new about themselves. Maybe leafy greens aren't as scary as they seem. Or (gasp) that they actually enjoy the refreshing feeling of basil touching their taste buds! Most important, they'll discover that trying new things, even something as simple as a few little green leaves grown from their garden, can be surprisingly fun.

Make It a Game: 15 points
Eat Your Colors: Green

Invite Exploration

Let your kids set up a taste test for another family member to try. Invite them to choose a variety of herbs that pique their interest. Have them create a series of questions to ask that start with the phrase, "I wonder . . ."

Nut-Free Basil Pesto

Nut-free basil pesto made straight from the garden is an easy addition to your garden-fresh menu. Most pesto recipes call for pine nuts, but this simple recipe has a creative twist: sunflower seeds. Our school is nut-free, so I am always looking for delicious and easy recipes that can be equally featured on our dinner and lunch menus. It's also super flexible. We tried our basil pesto on pasta and as a dip for our Tomato Pops (page 250). It's also tasty served with Simple Sautéed Chicken (page 283) or on a crusty French baguette.

PREP TIME: 5 minutes

Cook time: 0 minutes

Makes about 1 cup

INGREDIENTS:

1 cup packed fresh basil leaves

⅓ cup hulled roasted sunflower seeds

⅓ cup grated Parmesan cheese

1 clove garlic, minced

⅓ cup extra-virgin olive oil, plus more as needed

Kosher salt

DIRECTIONS:

1   Harvest your fresh basil. Wash it thoroughly and gently pat dry with paper towels.

2   Place the basil, sunflower seeds, Parmesan, and garlic in the bowl of a food processor. Process until the ingredients are well chopped, about 2 minutes.

3   Add the oil and process for another minute, or until smooth. Add salt to taste. For a smoother texture, add a little extra olive oil.

4   Enjoy with fresh pasta or as a dip for your veggies.

Tip *If you want to freeze your basil pesto, leave out the cheese. Portion the cheese-free pesto into an ice cube tray, cover, and freeze. Once frozen, remove the pesto cubes from the tray and store them in a glass container in the freezer. When you're ready to use your sauce, defrost a cube or two and add the grated Parmesan.*

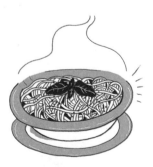

Cook Together

Beginners: Harvest the basil. Load the ingredients into the food processor.

Experts: Cut the veggies for dipping.

Basil Pesto Pizza

Homemade garden pizza is one of our favorite summertime meals—perfect for DIY dinner night. Pesto, made with fresh basil, gives this pizza a refreshing flavor. Encourage your kids to add fresh vegetables and herbs from your garden to personalize their pies.

PREP TIME: 15 minutes

WAIT TIME: 2 hours

COOK TIME: 20 minutes

Serves 4

INGREDIENTS:

½ recipe Whole Wheat Pizza Dough (page 119)

1 tablespoon extra-virgin olive oil

¼ cup Nut-Free Basil Pesto (page 230)

1 medium tomato, thinly sliced

¼ cup shredded mozzarella cheese

Torn fresh basil leaves, for garnish

DIRECTIONS:

1 Lightly oil a rimmed baking sheet. Press out the dough onto the baking sheet and set aside to rise until it doubles in size, about 2 hours.

2 Preheat the oven to 400°F. Brush the dough with the oil. Top evenly with the pesto and sliced tomatoes. Sprinkle with the cheese.

3 Bake for 15 to 20 minutes, or until the crust turns golden brown and the cheese has melted.

4 Top with basil leaves and serve.

Grow It

Our efforts to grow basil were consistently thwarted by slugs. It turns out they, too, love the taste of tender basil leaves. Friends recommended everything from sprinkling coffee grounds on the dirt surrounding the plant to strategically placing broken eggshells to defend our territory, but in the end, we found it easiest to simply plant our basil in pots, put them on our garden table, and call it a day. Place your pots in a sunny location that is easy for the kids to access, but not the slugs.

Simple Summer Peaches with Basil

Another easy way to try fresh basil is paired with sweet summer peaches. They make a great team.

PREP TIME: 5 minutes

COOK TIME: 0 minutes

Serves 4

INGREDIENTS:

5 peaches, pitted and cut into 1-inch pieces

1 tablespoon chopped fresh basil leaves

2 tablespoons fresh lemon juice (from 1 lemon)

Vanilla ice cream, for serving

DIRECTIONS:

1 In a medium bowl, combine the peaches, basil, and lemon juice. Toss gently to combine.

2 Serve with scoops of vanilla ice cream.

Fun Fact Basil is normally associated with Italian cooking, but it actually originated in India, where it was thought to ward off evil.

Buy in Season If you purchase basil from the farmers' market, trim the ends and place the stems in a small glass of water on your kitchen counter, like a bouquet. Basil does better at room temperature. The cold air of the refrigerator will turn the leaves black. Use within a few days.

Keep Trying Even if your kids don't like the taste of basil, enjoy the pleasures of growing it. Time spent together exploring and working in the garden is time well spent.

Explore Herbs: The Blind Taste Test

The Blind Taste Test is a fun way to break through when you hit the herb wall. I tried this experiment with micro greens, yet another source of foreign green flecks, but you can easily do the same experiment with fresh herbs from your garden, including basil.

"Which one tastes like bubblegum?" Like the jingle of the ice-cream truck, my question captured everyone's attention. Perched on our garden table were three small green mounds. Not sugar-coated candies, but tiny leaves no bigger than my daughter's thumbnail. With exuberant excitement, my new food explorers gathered around the table to uncover the mystery. The idea that a small green plant could taste like candy had them captivated.

Picking gingerly through the pile, little leaf by little leaf, they relished in the thrill of solving the puzzle. Shouts of incredulous discovery emerged. "I taste melon!" "This one tastes like cinnamon!" "You have to try this one! It takes like Froot Loops!"

Carried by their curiosity, I inquired, "How do you think the greens get their flavor?" The theories that emerged were intriguing. James's first hypothesis was that something was applied to the leaves in the same way that seasoning is applied to a flavorful dish. Catherine theorized that the leaves came from the baby version of a fruit or vegetable plant, like a lemon or a cucumber. Then together they toyed with the idea that the greens were grown in a garden with other fruits and vegetables, capturing their flavor through the soil. But the answer wasn't what I was after. It was their culinary curiosity that I celebrated.

Butter Lettuce

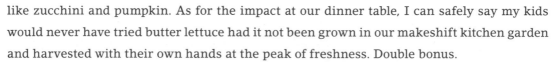

Next to herbs, butter lettuce is a busy mom's dream vegetable. Yes, you read that right. Lettuce is your friend. It is a simple crop to grow, which got us out into the garden, playing in the dirt. Like radishes, butter lettuce gave us the boost in confidence we needed to venture out and try to grow even more vegetables, like zucchini and pumpkin. As for the impact at our dinner table, I can safely say my kids would never have tried butter lettuce had it not been grown in our makeshift kitchen garden and harvested with their own hands at the peak of freshness. Double bonus.

Begin with starter plants, so that your garden can get rolling quickly. To avoid the leaves turning bitter during the hot summer months, plant your crop where the lettuce can take refuge in the shade and be sure to keep the soil moist. In addition to tender butter lettuce, encourage your kids to plant a variety of other lettuces including stiff, tall romaine and blushing, wispy looseleaf. Like members of a family, a range of personalities will make your garden much more interesting.

Let your kids harvest the lettuce and try it a few different ways. Dipping the tender leaves in a homemade vinaigrette is a simple strategy—many times more successful than trying to sell salad at our dinner table. It's also fun to use your homegrown lettuce as an alternative to bread, like a wrap. Leave a few of the heads to bolt, and let the seeds fall to the soil leaving treasure for the next season (and saving you some work). Most important, enjoy working in your garden together with your kids.

Make It a Game: 15 points
Eat Your Colors: Green

> ### Invite Exploration
> "How would you describe the taste of butter lettuce when it's freshly picked from the garden versus purchased from the grocery store?"

Chinese Chicken Wraps

When my mother-in-law, Sophia, arrives, she takes over the kitchen and there is never a complaint from the kids. They eat everything she makes! One of their favorite dishes is Chinese chicken, served up in fresh butter lettuce cups.

PREP TIME: 10 minutes

COOK TIME: 8 to 10 minutes

Serves 4

INGREDIENTS:

2 tablespoons grapeseed oil

½ cup diced carrots

½ cup diced celery

¼ cup diced water chestnuts

¼ cup diced mushrooms

2 cups diced Easy Roasted Chicken (page 282)

1 tablespoon tamari

1 green onion, diced

1 head butter lettuce

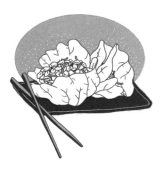

DIRECTIONS:

1   Heat a large wok over medium heat. Add the oil, then add the carrots and celery and sauté for 2 to 3 minutes, or until the vegetables begin to soften. Add the water chestnuts and mushrooms and sauté for 3 to 5 minutes more, or until the vegetables are lightly browned on the edges. Finally, add the cooked chicken and tamari. Toss to combine.

2   Transfer to a large serving bowl and garnish with the green onion. Serve family style, using the butter lettuce as wraps.

Cook Together

Beginners: Harvest the lettuce. Wash the lettuce.

Experts: Dice the vegetables. Sauté the vegetables.

Tip: To wash lettuce, fill a large bowl with cold water. Remove the damaged outer leaves. Place the remaining leaves in the water. Let the kids gently swish the leaves around with their hands. The dirt will settle to the bottom and the leaves will float. Remove the clean leaves and place on a towel to dry, or spin dry in a salad spinner.

Butter Lettuce Leaves with Simple Vinaigrette

My kids won't eat salad, but they are willing to dip tender butter lettuce leaves in a mild and simple dressing. This one does the trick. Experiment with fresh herbs from your garden to let your kids make their own mix.

PREP TIME: 5 minutes

COOK TIME: 0 minutes

Makes 1 cup

INGREDIENTS:

1 head butter lettuce

1 small clove garlic, minced

1 tablespoon red wine vinegar

¼ cup extra-virgin olive oil

2 tablespoons fresh lemon juice (from 1 lemon)

¼ teaspoon kosher salt

DIRECTIONS:

1 Harvest and wash your lettuce. Gently pat it dry with paper towels.

2 In a small bowl, combine the garlic, vinegar, oil, lemon juice, and salt.

3 Serve the dressing in little bowls and let your kids dip the lettuce leaves.

Tip *Whisk in a touch of Dijon mustard to give your dressing extra kick. Encourage your kids to taste as they mix. Does the dressing need more lemon? More salt?*

Grow It To start lettuce from seeds, fill the cups of an egg carton halfway with soil, sprinkle a few seeds in each section, then add a little more soil to cover. Water gently. Keep the egg carton in a sunny location, like a kitchen window. Sprouts will appear within a week or two. Once the seedlings have established leaves, transplant them to your garden.

Sunflower Butter Lettuce Wraps

Paired with sunflower butter or peanut butter, these wraps make a quick and tasty garden-fresh snack.

PREP TIME: 5 minutes

COOK TIME: 0 minutes

Makes 12 wraps

INGREDIENTS:

1 head butter lettuce

Sunflower butter

DIRECTIONS:

1 Harvest and wash your butter lettuce.

2 Keeping the leaves intact, spread 1 teaspoon of sunflower butter onto each piece of lettuce. Wrap and enjoy!

3 Then plant a new crop.

> **Keep Trying** Your kitchen garden is one of the keys to getting your kids to try new foods. When children grow their own food, they are more likely to try those foods. Encourage tasters as you tend.

Cucumbers

"No, thanks, I like cucumbers only when they are fresh-picked." Stating her case with a firm resolve, Catherine confidently passed the plate of cucumber sticks along to her brother. I didn't have a good comeback. How could I argue with her preference for fresh-picked veggies?

Some would say I should have encouraged an obligatory "no, thank you" bite—that acquiescing to Catherine's finicky stance on cucumbers would cause problems down the line. What would be next? Harvested at dawn to maintain their cool crispness?

After months of trying new foods together, I realized that Catherine truly experienced food in a more intense way than I did. Whether it's connected to her creative spirit or a physical trait that makes her taste things differently, it is something that I've come to recognize and honor. It's a part of her that I lovingly accept and *celebrate*.

My advice? When faced with peculiar pickiness at your table, remember that each person really can experience flavors, textures, and smells in different ways. And that taste buds grow and change, just like your kids. Definitely encourage lots of experimentation and tasters. But if someone draws a line in the soil after trying a food lots of different times, in lots of different ways, it's best to honor that line. Instead, focus on the fun of growing these foods, scouting them out at the farmers' market, and cooking them together.

Make It a Game: 10 points
Eat Your Colors: Green, Yellow/Orange

Invite Exploration

"How many different varieties of cucumber do you think we can find at the market?"

Asian Cucumber Salad

This easy cucumber salad is a homemade version of my favorite Japanese side dish. Five minutes delivers a tasty side to serve right away. Or put it back in the fridge to let the cucumbers brine—it's even better the second day, toted in a lunchbox with sesame noodles and mini chicken satays. Pair it with Pan-Seared Tofu Slices (page 288) for a quick and easy weeknight dinner. If, like Catherine and James, your kids turn up their noses at the vinegar, start by leaving it out. Work your way up in small portions.

PREP TIME: 5 minutes

Wait time: 15 minutes

Serves 4

INGREDIENTS:

1 large cucumber

¼ cup rice vinegar

1 teaspoon sugar

¼ teaspoon kosher salt

2 tablespoons sesame seeds

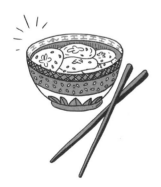

DIRECTIONS:

1   Using a potato peeler, let your kids peel the cucumber. Give it stripes like a zebra or peel off all the skin. Either way works well, so let your kids decide.

2   Using a small paring knife, cut the peeled cucumber into thin slices—the thinner the better. Set the slices aside in a medium bowl. Discard the ends.

3   In a small bowl, whisk together the vinegar, sugar, and salt until combined and the sugar is fully dissolved. Add the vinegar mixture to the cucumbers, sprinkle on the sesame seeds, and toss gently to coat.

4   Cover and refrigerate for 15 minutes to let the flavors meld.

5   Serve cold.

Cook Together

Beginners: Peel the cucumber. Whisk the dressing. Add the sprinkles.

Experts: Cut the cucumber.

Tip: One of my go-to kitchen tools is a simple potato peeler. We use it for preparing everything from potatoes and apples to zucchini and cucumber. Look for one with a rubber grip and a blade that is perpendicular to the handle (making a T shape). I've found this style easiest to use with my kids.

Minty Cucumber Salad

This Mediterranean-style salad makes a quick, no-cook side dish for hot summer days. Pair it with grilled chicken satays, fresh veggies, toasted whole wheat pita, and hummus.

PREP TIME: 10 minutes

COOK TIME: 0 minutes

Serves 4

INGREDIENTS:

3 large cucumbers

1 cup nonfat plain yogurt

2 tablespoons extra-virgin olive oil

1 tablespoon coarsely chopped fresh mint leaves

1 tablespoon fresh lemon juice (from ½ lemon)

Kosher salt

DIRECTIONS:

1 Peel the cucumbers and slice them into ¼-inch cubes. Set aside.

2 In a large bowl, whisk together the yogurt, oil, mint, and lemon juice.

3 Combine the cucumbers with the yogurt-mint dressing. Season with kosher salt to taste.

4 Serve immediately.

Grow It

Cucumbers grow best in the warm summer sun. Experiment with different varieties in your kitchen garden. Lemon cucumbers are a favorite—shaped like an apple, they are a little more sweet than regular cucumbers.

Cucumber Tea Sandwiches

Take the edge off hot summer afternoons with cool and crisp cucumber sandwiches. Serve with a batch of homemade Lavender Lemonade (page 271).

PREP TIME: 10 minutes

COOK TIME: 0 minutes

Serves 4

INGREDIENTS:

1 large cucumber

8 slices whole wheat bread

4 tablespoons whipped cream cheese, plus more for serving

4 teaspoons honey

Lavender Lemonade (page 271) or Lavender Mint Tea (page 272), for serving

DIRECTIONS:

1 Peel and slice the cucumber into ¼-inch wheels. Set aside.

2 Place the slices of bread on a cutting board. Spread 1 tablespoon of cream cheese on each slice. Top each slice with 4 slices of cucumber and drizzle with 1 teaspoon of honey.

3 Top with the remaining 4 slices of bread. Using a round cookie cutter, cut the sandwich into circles. Discard the crusts.

4 Top with a pea-size dollop of cream cheese and a small slice of cucumber. Serve with Lavender Lemonade or Lavender Mint Tea.

Keep Trying Another fun way to try cucumber is to make flavored water. Chop a cucumber into ¼-inch pieces. Place the pieces in an ice cube tray, fill with water, and freeze. Drop the cubes into your water for a refreshing, cucumber-infused summer sipper. Bonus: It's a great way to stay hydrated on hot summer days.

Green Onions

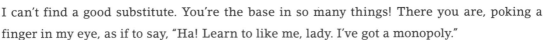

Drat you, onions! Why are you so hard to like? I've tried everything, and my daughter still picks at you. The worst part is that I can't find a good substitute. You're the base in so many things! There you are, poking a finger in my eye, as if to say, "Ha! Learn to like me, lady. I've got a monopoly."

I've chopped onions into the finest mince, barely noticeable to the human eye. I've simmered onions down to their softest touch to dull the sharp edge of their flavor. But Catherine can spot the faintest hint of them. The reality is, I still use them, for how could a flavorful chicken soup be made in their absence, but I navigate around them when serving Catherine. Instead of admitting defeat, I looked for the silver lining (there always has to be one, right?). There remain a few reasons to like onions, even with their attitude.

First, onions are a great way to practice chopping. The irony is that while Catherine won't eat onions, she's the first to dice them! She lights a votive to keep away the tears, and happily dices for any recipe that calls for an onion base—great practice for her knife skills. It may not be onions, but it's highly likely that you have a similar food nemesis in your family. Remember: Even if they don't eat it, they are benefiting from the experience of cooking it. There is learning, just maybe not the learning you planned.

Second, onions are easy to grow, and they make a welcome addition to our kitchen garden each spring. Our preference is for green onions, aka scallions, because they don't require much maintenance and they work particularly well in container gardens. Their milder flavor is also easier for kids to warm up to.

Make It a Game: 15 points
Eat Your Colors: White, Green

> ### Invite Exploration
> "Why onions make you cry? What could we do to stop our eyes from tearing?"

Green Onion Pancakes

Green onion pancakes are the only exception to Catherine's longstanding onion boycott. They are delicious alongside a steamy bowl of noodles. Next to gobbling up these savory pancakes, kneading and rolling the dough is the best part of this recipe for my kids.

PREP TIME: 15 minutes

Wait time: 30 minutes

COOK TIME: 25 minutes

Serves 6

INGREDIENTS:

2 cups whole wheat all-purpose flour

¾ cup boiling water

½ teaspoon kosher salt

3 tablespoons grapeseed oil, plus more for brushing

8 green onions, green parts only, finely chopped

Ginger–Green Onion Dipping Sauce (page 244), for serving

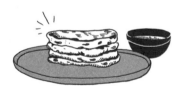

DIRECTIONS:

1 In a large bowl, combine the flour, water, and salt until it forms a ball. Set aside to cool.

2 Working on a lightly floured wooden cutting board, knead the cooled dough gently until it's smooth and elastic, about 10 minutes. Depending on the age of your children, it may be easier to divide the dough into quarters before kneading, then recombine before Step 3. Grease your kids' hands with a little bit of grapeseed oil before you get started to avoid the dough sticking to their fingers.

3 Transfer the ball back to the bowl and cover, leaving a small section uncovered to allow the gases to escape. Let stand for 30 minutes.

4 Form the dough into a log, then slice it into 24 rounds. Using a rolling pin, roll out each circle on the cutting board. Brush with grapeseed oil, sprinkle with green onions (about 1 teaspoon), and roll the pancake up like a rug with

Cook Together

Beginners: Knead and roll the dough. Form the pancakes.

Experts: Chop the green onions.

Tip: Don't worry about perfectly shaped pancakes. Let your kids take the lead and experiment with different shapes and sizes. This is a great family cooking project because you don't need to be exact!

the green onions tucked inside. Then roll the cylinder into a coil, like a cinnamon roll. Flatten the roll into a pancake with a rolling pin or the palm of your hand. Green onions should be peeking out all over.

5 Heat a large frying pan over medium-high heat. Add 1 tablespoon of grapeseed oil and 4 of the onion pancakes. Cook for 2 to 3 minutes, or until golden brown, then flip and cook the other side for 2 to 3 minutes more. Transfer to a paper towel–lined plate to drain and cool. Repeat, refreshing the oil in between batches.

6 Cut the pancakes into quarters and serve warm, with Ginger–Green Onion Dipping Sauce.

Ginger–Green Onion Dipping Sauce

PREP TIME: 5 minutes
COOK TIME: 1 minute
Makes ¼ cup

INGREDIENTS:

½ teaspoon grapeseed oil

½ teaspoon finely chopped peeled fresh ginger

½ teaspoon sesame oil

3 tablespoons tamari or soy sauce

2 green onions, green parts only, finely chopped

DIRECTIONS:

1 Heat a small frying pan over medium heat. Add the grapeseed oil, ginger, and sesame oil and sauté for 1 minute, or until the ginger is fragrant.

2 Remove the pan from the heat, add the tamari, and stir to combine.

3 In a small bowl, pour the sizzling ginger-tamari mixture over the green onions. Serve warm in small dipping bowls, alongside your Green Onion Pancakes (pages 243).

Grow It A green onion's flavor gets stronger as it grows. For a mild flavor, harvest green onions when the slender green leaves are young, or about 6 inches tall.

Green Onion and Mushroom Omelet

A simple breakfast dish, this omelet is a gentle way to introduce green onions to your kids. Add more or less green onion depending on their preference. If they're feeling adventurous, add other seasonal veggies like asparagus.

PREP TIME: 10 minutes

COOK TIME: 10 minutes

Serves 4

INGREDIENTS:

2 tablespoons extra-virgin olive oil, plus more as needed

6 green onions, green parts only, finely chopped, plus more for garnish

1 cup cremini mushroom slices (about ¼ inch thick)

6 large eggs, lightly beaten

½ cup shredded mozzarella cheese

DIRECTIONS:

1 Heat a medium frying pan over medium heat. Add the oil, green onions, and mushrooms and cook for 3 minutes, or until the mushrooms release their juices and turn golden brown. Add extra oil if the mushrooms stick to the pan.

2 Pour the eggs over the green onion–mushroom mixture. Stir gently to combine. Reduce the heat to low, cover, and let simmer for 5 minutes, or until the bottom of the omelet is golden brown. Partway through cooking, lift the edges of the omelet and let some of the uncooked egg run into the bottom of the pan.

3. Flip the omelet, add the cheese, and cook for 2 minutes more. To serve, fold in half, slice into quarters, and garnish with extra green onions.

Tip *To easily flip the omelet, use a spatula to loosen the edges of the egg. Place a heatproof plate on top of the pan. Carefully turn the pan over, holding the plate in place. Use the spatula to slide the omelet back into the pan to cook the second side.*

Keep Trying Even if your kids won't eat onions, always invite them to chop them for your recipes. Try different strategies—like lighting a votive—to see what works best to hold back the tears. Frame it as a good opportunity to work on their knife skills. The more familiar they become with any food, including onions, the more likely they will be to try it.

Radishes

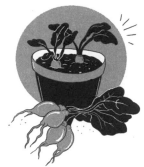

Growing radishes is like riding a bike with training wheels. For beginners like my kids and me, they make it easy to get rolling and you quickly feel the thrill of growing your own food. Sprouts appear a few short days after planting the seeds, and within a month you've got a batch of blushing beauties ready to be pulled up from the ground. Those training wheels were exactly what I needed when we started experimenting with growing our own food: an easy win.

When it came time to eat our radishes, we started simply by sampling them raw. Catherine spent a weekend morning gingerly slicing our garden-fresh radishes into delicate, wafer-thin layers and artfully arranging her creations on a tiny tasting platter for everyone to enjoy. Then we moved to cooking. Drawing inspiration from Deborah Madison, author of eleven cookbooks including one of my current favorites, *Vegetable Literacy*, we gathered a few more ingredients from our garden, supplemented them with finds from the farmers' market, and together we experimented with how to cook radishes, leaves and all. Radish presents another fun opportunity to use the whole plant—its frilly, dark green leaves are edible, too.

My kids are certainly not ravenous for radishes—that I wouldn't expect from a first encounter—but I was happy that they were at least willing to give it a try and that radishes helped build that all-important confidence to continue trying to grow (some) of our own food. As you start experimenting with your kitchen garden, I'd highly recommend adding radishes to your list. They are the easy win that will get your efforts off to a solid start.

Make It a Game: 15 points
Eat Your Colors: Red

Invite Exploration

"How do you think the French Breakfast radish got its name?"

Sautéed Radish Salad

This is a great example of a garden-to-table dish. Quick and easy. Do not leave the vegetables in the pan too long, or they will wilt from the heat. Just a quick flash in the pan is all they need.

PREP TIME: 10 minutes

COOK TIME: 5 minutes

Serves 4

INGREDIENTS:

3 to 4 small radishes, leaves on

1 tablespoon extra-virgin olive oil

½ cup shelled English peas

1 tablespoon fresh lemon juice (from ½ lemon)

Kosher salt

DIRECTIONS:

1 Wash and prepare your vegetables. Gather as much as you can from your garden. Round out your recipe with fresh veggies from the farmers' market. Slice the radishes into quarters. Coarsely chop the leaves.

2 Heat a large frying pan over medium heat. Add the oil, then the radishes. Sauté for 2 to 3 minutes, or until the radishes soften slightly.

3 Add the peas and the radish leaves. Add a touch of water at this point if you need to. Continue to sauté for 1 to 2 minutes more, or until the radish leaves have wilted.

4 Before serving, toss the vegetables with the lemon juice and kosher salt to taste.

Recipe inspired by Deborah Madison, author of Vegetable Literacy.

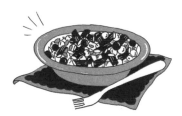

Cook Together

Beginners: Harvest the radishes. Shell the peas. Squeeze the lemon juice.

Experts: Slice the vegetables.

Tip: Radishes are relatively easy to slice. Let your kids use them to practice their knife skills. Encourage them to try making lots of different patterns.

Quick-Pickled Radishes

Pickling is another tasty way to enjoy your bounty of radishes. Invite your kids to try this method with a variety of summer vegetables, including a few new foods like okra and cucumber.

PREP TIME: 10 minutes

COOK TIME: 5 minutes

Serves 4

INGREDIENTS:

1 bunch radishes (about 1 pound)

1 cup vinegar

1 tablespoon honey

2 cloves garlic

½ teaspoon kosher salt

DIRECTIONS:

1 Wash and cut the radishes into quarters or slices. Discard the leaves. Place the cut radishes into a large mason jar.

2 In a small saucepan over medium heat, combine the vinegar, honey, garlic, salt, and 1 cup water. Bring to a boil, then reduce the heat and simmer for 2 minutes, or until the liquid forms a thin syrup.

3 Pour the hot liquid over the radishes. Cool to room temperature, then cover the jar and refrigerate for 24 hours before serving.

Buy in Season There are so many wonderful varieties of radishes that will appear at your farmers' market, and there is a special one for each season. In winter, look for watermelon radishes, with their pale green exterior and vibrant pink interior. In summer, seek out the French Breakfast radish—its long slender fingers look like they've been dipped in cream.

Grow It The flavor of radishes change as fast as they grow—they are tender but become harsh as time passes. That difference in flavor captured Catherine and James and contributed to their willingness to give radishes a try. Experiment with growing a few different types of radishes, including fast-growing spring radishes and varieties that take longer to mature, like daikon.

Keep Trying Radishes make a great predinner snack, just like carrots and celery. Serve them raw or pickled along with Healthy Homemade Hummus (page 278). Let your kids lightly dip radish wedges in salt for another flavor sensation. The more often they see this vegetable on your table (and in your garden), the more willing they will be to give it a try.

Cherry Tomatoes

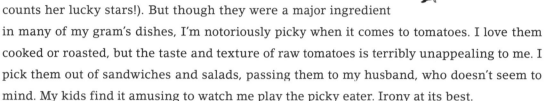

Growing up in an Italian family, you'd think that tomatoes would be one of my favorite foods, by nature or nurture. My gram cooked for our family each week—hand-cut ravioli with tomato sauce, homemade minestrone soup, and frittata (my mom still counts her lucky stars!). But though they were a major ingredient in many of my gram's dishes, I'm notoriously picky when it comes to tomatoes. I love them cooked or roasted, but the taste and texture of raw tomatoes is terribly unappealing to me. I pick them out of sandwiches and salads, passing them to my husband, who doesn't seem to mind. My kids find it amusing to watch me play the picky eater. Irony at its best.

Then the tomatoes we planted in our kitchen garden changed everything.

For me, the flavor of peak-season, garden-grown tomatoes is completely different (and wildly more appealing) than the mushy, tasteless slices that attempt to pawn themselves off as tomatoes at other times of the year. My kids feel the same way, and are much more willing to try cherry tomatoes plucked from the vine and juicy heirlooms from the local farmers' market, when they appear for a brief spell in late summer.

Tomatoes are a prime example of how modern industrial efforts have failed us. Big&Co may have engineered tomatoes to make the trek through our complicated food system without a hint of bruising. But what they gained in transportability they gave up in flavor. In this case, pickiness pays big dividends when it comes to pleasing the palate.

Make It a Game: 5 points
Eat Your Colors: Yellow/Orange, Red

Invite Exploration

"What do you notice about tomatoes that are freshly picked from the garden versus tomatoes you find at the grocery store?"

Tomato Pops

Caprese salad with a kid-friendly twist! These pint-size tomato-mozzarella skewers make fresh-picked cherry tomatoes even more fun (and easy) to enjoy! Serve up your Tomato Pops with a side of Nut-Free Basil Pesto (page 230) and let everyone enjoy giving their pops a dip!

PREP TIME: 10 minutes

COOK TIME: 0 minutes

Serves 4

INGREDIENTS:

1 pint cherry tomatoes

1 cup mozzarella balls or cubes of your favorite cheese

¼ cup extra-virgin olive oil

Kosher salt

Handful fresh basil leaves

12 wooden skewers

DIRECTIONS:

1 Wash the tomatoes and, using your fingers, remove the green tops. Load the tomatoes into a large bowl as you go.

2 Drain the mozzarella balls, then add them to the tomatoes.

3 Add the oil and salt to the tomatoes and mozzarella. Stir gently to combine.

4 Skewer the tomatoes, mozzarella, and basil leaves, alternating between them.

5 Serve the skewers in a small glass vase or cup, like a bouquet. Mix together the remaining ingredients into a fresh Caprese salad.

Cook Together

Beginners: Harvest the tomatoes. Mix the ingredients. Load up the skewers.

Tip: This recipe is easy enough for kids of all ages to make. Invite them to create their own patterns on the skewers.

Cherry Tomato Boats with Hummus and Parsley

Kids love appetizers, too, and these little red gems are the ticket. Place them out on the counter and let your kids nibble and nosh as you're making dinner together.

PREP TIME: 10 minutes

COOK TIME: 0 minutes

Serves 4

INGREDIENTS:

1 pint cherry tomatoes

½ cup Healthy Homemade Hummus (page 278)

Fresh parsley, for garnish

DIRECTIONS:

1 Wash the tomatoes and, using your fingers, remove their green tops. Using a paring knife, halve the tomatoes from top to tip.

2 Using a small spoon, scoop out the insides of the tomatoes and discard.

3 Fill each tomato boat with hummus and top with a sprig of fresh parsley.

4 Serve immediately.

Buy in Season Invite your kids to find a range of tomato varieties at the farmers' market. Heirlooms are beautiful with their watercolor-like patterns. Baskets of yellow, orange, and red cherry tomatoes make for a colorful salad. Ask the farmer, "Which is your favorite variety of tomato, and why?"

Grow It Start from small plants as opposed to seeds. Provide a sunny location and a trellis to grow on. Once your tomatoes take hold, they'll need space to stretch their vines. Plant your colors: Sungold (yellow), Early Cherry (red), and Fruity Orange (orange).

Roasted Cherry Tomatoes

Roasting not only changes the flavor and texture of tomatoes, it makes it easier to absorb the antioxidants packed inside.[1] This simple side dish is delicious paired with Sesame-Crusted Salmon (page 224), Easy Roasted Chicken (page 282), or atop a garden-fresh pizza.

PREP TIME: 10 minutes

COOK TIME: 20 minutes

Serves 4

INGREDIENTS:

2 pints cherry tomatoes (stems removed)

1 tablespoon extra-virgin olive oil

¼ teaspoon kosher salt

DIRECTIONS:

1 Preheat the oven to 400°F.

2 On a rimmed baking sheet, combine the tomatoes, oil, and salt.

3 Bake for 20 minutes, or until the tomatoes are soft and slightly charred.

Tip You can cut the tomatoes in half, if you prefer.

Keep Trying Even Harvard University's head of nutrition, Dr. Walter Willett, needed time to warm up to tomatoes! When I asked Dr. Willett which food he likes now but didn't as a child, and what helped him make that change, he emphatically replied, "Tomatoes. Olive oil and basil helped."

Gram's Homemade Tomato Sauce

Making homemade sauce is a wonderful Sunday afternoon activity. It makes the whole house smell delicious. What I love about this recipe is that you can make it ahead and enjoy the fruits of your labor in different dishes all week long. The sauce can be used for dressing homemade pizza, pasta, and chicken dishes. To save time, this recipe uses boxed chopped tomatoes. Add a few handfuls of garden-fresh tomatoes at the end to give this sauce a seasonal touch.

PREP TIME: 20 minutes

COOK TIME: about 2 hours

Serves 16 to 20

INGREDIENTS:

5 (28-ounce) boxes chopped Italian tomatoes

1 (28-ounce) jar tomato juice

1 tablespoon extra-virgin olive oil

1 tablespoon unsalted butter

1 slice pancetta, cut into ½-inch pieces

3 slices extra-thin prosciutto

½ large white onion, finely chopped

3 cloves garlic, finely chopped

1 medium shallot, finely chopped

½ teaspoon marjoram

1 teaspoon sugar

Kosher salt and freshly ground black pepper

A few handfuls of fresh basil and parsley

DIRECTIONS:

1 Over a large bowl, run the tomatoes through a food mill with the finest attachment. (Gram was adamant about removing all of the seeds from the tomatoes.)

2 Add tomato juice to the strained tomatoes. Set aside.

3 In a large stockpot, heat the oil and butter over medium-high heat. Add the pancetta and fry until crispy, then remove and discard. Add the prosciutto and fry until crispy.

4 Reduce the heat slightly, then add the onions, garlic, and shallots and sauté for 3 to 5 minutes, or until the onions are soft and translucent. Add the marjoram and sugar to the onion mixture and stir well to combine.

5 Add the tomato mixture to the pot. Lightly season with salt and pepper. Bring to a strong boil, then reduce the heat to low and simmer, partially covered, for at least 2 hours, stirring frequently. Wipe the water from the lid of the pot several times throughout to remove condensation. The sauce will reduce by about half.

6 Stir in a handful of parsley and a few sprigs of basil.

7 Let the sauce cool, then portion it into glass containers. Save some for use during the week and freeze the rest. It can be stored in your freezer for up to 3 months. (If freezing sauce, do not use glass containers.)

Tip *If you're lucky enough to have fresh tomatoes from your garden, chop them into ½-inch dice and add a cup or two to the sauce during the last 20 minutes of simmering. This is a great way to add fresh, seasonal veggies to your delicious, homemade sauce.*

corn

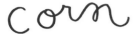

When corn arrives at the farmers' market, it makes my heart sing. Late summer rolling into early fall is my favorite time of year, and fat ears of fresh corn, stacked high on rickety wooden tables, are an enduring hallmark of the season. Grilled corn with a kiss of butter ranks high on our list of family favorites.

But corn can get a really bad rap. It's the archenemy in the obesity crisis (high-fructose corn syrup in our soda), it causes problems for our food supply (cornfed cattle), and it tops the charts when it comes to genetically modified foods (second only to soybeans).[2] For all of these reasons, corn can be a problem. But as with many things, each problem presents an opportunity. With corn, it was the opportunity to talk with my kids about how to choose wisely.

We discussed the differences between fresh-picked corn, grown organically by a local farmer, and corn that is added to processed foods to make it sweeter (or more convenient)—the corn you eat when you're looking (on the cob) versus when you're not looking (in processed foods). Corn comes in many forms, and the trick is figuring out how to spot it so you know what you're eating (see page 39).

When corn season arrives, take the opportunity to enjoy it with your kids. Talk about the myriad ways that corn is used in our food system and how to find it on a food label. Above all else, enjoy corn in one of the simplest and most pleasurable ways—sourced from a local, certified organic farmer and eaten straight from the cob.

Make It a Game: 10 points
Eat Your Colors: Yellow/Orange, Red

Invite Exploration

"What are some ways we can tell if produce is grown organically?"

Garlic Corn

This is one of our favorite ways to enjoy sweet, late-summer corn. Apart from the delicious flavor, the best part of this recipe for my kids is shucking the fresh corn. Toss in a few chopped tomatoes for a colorful variation.

PREP TIME: 10 minutes

COOK TIME: 7 minutes

Serves 4

INGREDIENTS:

2 large ears fresh corn

1 tablespoon unsalted butter

¼ teaspoon garlic powder

Kosher salt, to taste

Fresh parsley, for garnish

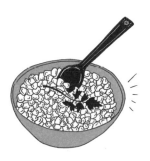

DIRECTIONS:

1 Remove the husks and silks from the corn. Discard.

2 Break the cobs in half, then place the flat end of the cob on a cutting board and slice the kernels from the cob.

3 In a large frying pan, melt the butter over medium heat. Once it is bubbling, but before it starts to turn brown, add the corn kernels. Simmer gently for 5 to 7 minutes, or until the edges of the kernels turn golden.

4 Add the garlic powder to the corn and stir to combine. Add salt to taste.

5 Garnish with fresh parsley. Serve warm.

Tip Add ½ cup of diced tomatoes for an extra pop of color.

Cook Together

Beginners: Remove the husks. Season the dish.

Experts: Cut the kernels from the cob. Sauté the corn.

Tip: Set up your prep station outside, so that your kids can work freely and corn silks don't litter your floor.

Easy Corn Salsa

This simple salsa is another fun way to enjoy sweet summer corn. It's a great side for DIY dinner night, paired with Black Bean Burritos (page 172). Use this recipe as a base, and encourage your kids to add more colorful foods to make their own mix.

PREP TIME: 10 minutes

COOK TIME: 5 minutes

Makes 1½ to 2 cups

INGREDIENTS:

2 large ears fresh corn

½ cup chopped tomatoes

2 tablespoons fresh lime juice (from 1 lime)

½ teaspoon finely chopped garlic

¼ teaspoon kosher salt

1 tablespoon coarsely chopped fresh cilantro leaves

DIRECTIONS:

1 Bring a large pot of water to a boil.

2 Remove the husks and silks from the corn and discard. Add the corn to the boiling water and cook for 3 to 5 minutes, or until the kernels are bright yellow. Remove and rinse with cold water.

3 Working over a large bowl, cut the kernels from the cob. Discard the cobs. Add the tomatoes, lime juice, garlic, salt, and cilantro. Stir gently to combine.

4 Cover and refrigerate for 15 minutes to let the flavors meld before serving.

Popping Corn on the Cob

Our friends the Levenbergs introduced us to this fun way to make popcorn. At harvest time, head out to a local farm that grows corn. Call ahead to be sure they grow popping corn—it's a special variety. Pick your corn, then take it home, place the whole ear (husk and all) into a brown paper bag, and let it dry completely. You'll know it's ready when the husks are flaky. If you pick your corn in the early fall, the cobs should be ready by about Thanksgiving. Then make popcorn!

PREP TIME: 0 minutes

COOK TIME: 2 minutes

Makes about 2 cups per cob

INGREDIENTS:

1 ear dried popping corn, husks removed

Kosher salt

Unsalted butter, melted

DIRECTIONS:

1 Place one dried cob in a brown paper bag. Fold the bag down 2 or 3 times to keep the popped corn inside the bag.

2 Microwave the bag for 2 minutes on high.

3 Transfer the popped corn to a large bowl. Season with kosher salt and a little melted butter. Enjoy with friends.

Buy in Season Organic corn will almost always have a few kernels missing from the tip of the cob. Without pesticides, corn earworms can nestle into the husks and eat away at your fresh corn. If you peel back a husk to find one of these critters, don't worry. Just discard the worm, cut off the eaten section, and wash thoroughly before cooking.

Okra

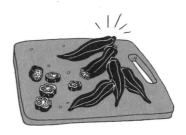

In my mind, there's really not much to like about okra. It's slimy. It's hairy. Its seeds get caught in your teeth. Can you tell I'm not a fan? You'd think that because of my reluctance, my kids wouldn't like it, either, but they do. Surprisingly, the biggest okra fan in our house is Catherine. It's her go-to green. Why she loves this strange vegetable and not others that seem much easier to enjoy (like celery) is a mystery.

Okra first made an appearance on our table when Catherine was a toddler. But I found it tremendously challenging to prepare this particular vegetable in a way that was appealing for me. The only (marginally) tolerable recipe I used was risotto—in risotto, its sliminess was masked for me. Luckily, my husband, Anthony, kept at it despite my pickiness, stir-frying okra or roasting it whenever we found it at the local market. *Fine for them to eat it*, I thought, *but not me!*

Then Catherine called me on it.

"You should give it another try, Mom. Maybe you'll like it this time."

Oh, how the tables had turned! Listening to my own advice played back to me, how could I not take it? With a slight quiver, I tried the okra. I try it each time it arrives on our table. I'm still not a fan, but what's important is walking the walk. If I want my kids to be flexible and open to trying new things, even when they think they have made a firm decision, then I need to be that way, too. Like it or not, your kids are watching your every move, so model good behavior, including trying okra (even when you don't like it!).

Make It a Game: 15 points
Eat Your Colors: Green

Invite Exploration

"What adjectives would you use to describe okra?"

Okra Risotto

Okra is packed with goodness, particularly vitamin C and fiber. It's also relatively inexpensive and in plentiful supply at farmers' markets in the summer, which means there's even more reason to give it a try. For me, adding okra to risotto is the easiest way to bring out the best in this vegetable (and cover up some of its less desirable qualities, namely sliminess).

PREP TIME: 10 minutes

COOK TIME: 15 minutes

Serves 4

INGREDIENTS:

½ pound okra

4 cups Chicken Broth (page 99)

2 tablespoons unsalted butter

2 tablespoons extra-virgin olive oil

1 small onion, finely chopped

1 cup arborio rice

½ cup white wine

½ cup grated Parmesan cheese

Kosher salt

Cook Together

Beginners: Wash and trim the okra. Stir the risotto.

Experts: Cut the vegetables.

DIRECTIONS:

1 Wash the okra and cut the pods into ½-inch pieces. You should have about 2 cups. Set aside.

2 In a medium saucepan, bring the broth to a boil, then reduce the heat to low to keep the broth warm.

3 In a large sauté pan, melt the butter into the oil over low to medium heat. Add the onion and sauté for 2 to 3 minutes, or until the onion is soft and translucent. Add the rice and stir frequently until the edges of the grains are transparent, 3 to 4 minutes.

4 Using a measuring cup, pour 2 cups of warm broth over the rice and stir until absorbed, about 10 minutes. Add the remaining broth and the white wine and continue stirring for 5 minutes more. Be sure the bottom of the pan doesn't dry out.

5 Add the okra and continue cooking for 5 minutes more, or until most of the liquid has been absorbed, the rice is cooked but firm, and some liquid remains.

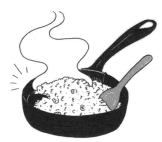

6 Stir in the Parmesan and season with salt before serving.

Simple Sautéed Okra

This recipe is Catherine's favorite way to enjoy okra. It's simple and quick, making it an easy way to add color to your table on a weeknight. Pair it with Simple Sautéed Chicken (page 283) or Sesame-Crusted Salmon (page 224).

PREP TIME: 5 minutes

COOK TIME: 7 minutes

Serves 4

INGREDIENTS:

½ pound okra

1 tablespoon extra-virgin olive oil

Kosher salt

DIRECTIONS:

1 Wash the okra and cut the pods into ½-inch pieces. You should have about 2 cups.

2 Heat a large sauté pan over medium-high heat. Add 1 tablespoon of extra-virgin olive oil and then the okra. Cook for 5 to 7 minutes, or until the okra is browned on the edges.

3 Season with salt before serving.

Buy in Season Pick small green pods that are about two inches long.

Garlic-Roasted Okra

Roasting okra is another easy way to prepare this vegetable. Try it with a variety of seasonings—garlic powder, cumin, and paprika are great options.

PREP TIME: 5 minutes

COOK TIME: 15 minutes

Serves 4

INGREDIENTS:

1 pound okra

2 tablespoons extra-virgin olive oil

½ teaspoon garlic salt

DIRECTIONS:

1 Preheat the oven to 400°F.

2 Wash and trim the okra. Set the pods on a paper towel and pat completely dry, removing any excess water.

3 In a large bowl, toss the okra with the oil and garlic salt until thoroughly coated.

4 Place the okra on a rimmed baking sheet and roast for 15 minutes, tossing occasionally in the pan to ensure even roasting. The okra should be nicely browned and fork-tender (but not mushy).

5 Serve immediately.

Peaches

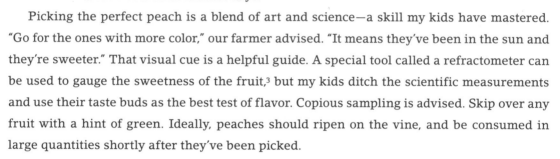

A sweet peach is something to behold. The gentle curves and soft, velvet skin makes a peach as much fun to cradle in the palm of your hand as it is to eat. And eat them we do, in large quantities. When peaches arrive at the farmers' market, my kids race to taste every delicious variety they can find—those samples serve as their breakfast on summer market days.

Picking the perfect peach is a blend of art and science—a skill my kids have mastered. "Go for the ones with more color," our farmer advised. "It means they've been in the sun and they're sweeter." That visual cue is a helpful guide. A special tool called a refractometer can be used to gauge the sweetness of the fruit,[3] but my kids ditch the scientific measurements and use their taste buds as the best test of flavor. Copious sampling is advised. Skip over any fruit with a hint of green. Ideally, peaches should ripen on the vine, and be consumed in large quantities shortly after they've been picked.

While peaches are perfect simply sliced, they also provide a fun and easy way to cook with your kids. In our house, James is the master of homemade peach ice cream. Predictably, a line forms outside our front door on the days he's making a batch. Grilling peaches is another way to try this simple sweet fruit—toss them on the grill with your portobellos and fresh corn. And if you're lucky, your local farmer might have a basket of overripe peaches that he's selling at a discount. Load up and make peach fruit leather—yet another fun recipe to cook together with your kids.

Make It a Game: 5 points
Eat Your Colors: Yellow/Orange

Invite Exploration

"Which foods do you think pair well with peaches?"

Grilled Peaches

Grilling peaches dials up their sweetness even further and makes a delicious dessert. Plus, grilling is an easy way to try familiar foods, especially fruit, in a new way. My kids love the challenge of making a whole meal, dessert included, on the grill!

PREP TIME: 5 minutes

COOK TIME: 6 to 8 minutes

Serves 4

INGREDIENTS:

4 small peaches, ripe but firm

1 tablespoon extra-virgin olive oil

Vanilla ice cream and honey, for serving

Cook Together

Beginners: Paint the peaches with olive oil.

Experts: Grill the peaches.

DIRECTIONS:

1 Preheat a grill to medium heat.

2 Slice the peaches in half and remove the pits. Using a pastry brush, paint both sides of the fruit with oil.

3 Grill the peaches cut-side down for 3 to 4 minutes. Turn the fruit and cook for 3 to 4 minutes more, or until the skin has light grill marks and the fruit is heated through.

4 Serve warm. Add scoops of vanilla ice cream and a drizzle of honey for an extra treat.

Tip *Choose smaller fruit for grilling. Larger fruit tends to burn before heating all the way through.*

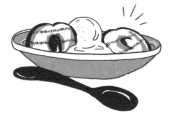

Easy Peach Ice Cream

James is the ice-cream expert in our house. He learned this recipe from his auntie Suzanne, one of our favorite family chefs. It reminds us of our carefree summer vacations together, and the pleasures of a simple, homemade treat enjoyed with friends and family.

PREP TIME: 10 minutes

WAIT TIME: 4 hours

Serves 6

INGREDIENTS:

1 pound peaches

⅓ cup sugar

½ teaspoon pure vanilla extract

¾ cup heavy cream

Fresh blackberries, for garnish

DIRECTIONS:

1 Peel and slice the peaches into ½-inch thick wedges. Place the wedges in a single layer on a parchment paper–lined rimmed baking sheet. Freeze until solid, about 4 hours.

2 Transfer the frozen peaches to a food processor with the sugar and process for 1 minute until the mixture looks like snow.

3 With the machine running, add the vanilla and cream. Process for 2 minutes, or until the mixture is smooth and creamy.

4 Serve immediately with fresh blackberries. This ice cream is best enjoyed right away.

Tip To easily peel peaches, gently place them in boiling water for 30 seconds, then give them a bath in ice water. Once they are cool, invite your kids to peel away the skins.

Buy in Season Head out to the farmers' market together and pick up a bushel of fresh peaches. Ask the farmer how to find the best of the bunch, how they like to prepare them, and what new varieties they are growing this season. Circle back the next week to share what you made. Use peaches as an opportunity to get to know your farmer.

Peach Fruit Leather

This is the perfect recipe for overripe peaches. It is one of our lunchbox favorites. Be sure the puree isn't spread too thin, otherwise, your fruit leather will be too crispy and won't roll properly. Double the batch and make enough to share with friends. Everyone will want to trade lunches with you.

PREP TIME: 5 minutes

COOK TIME: 3 to 4 hours

Serves 4

INGREDIENTS:

4 peaches, pitted but skin left on

1 tablespoon honey

DIRECTIONS:

1 Preheat the oven to 150°F. Line a rimmed baking sheet with parchment paper.

2 In a food processor, combine the peaches, honey, and ¼ cup water. Process for 2 minutes, or until smooth.

3 Pour the mixture onto the lined baking sheet and spread it evenly with a spoon.

4 Let dry in the oven for 3 to 4 hours, or until the fruit is a little bit tacky.

5 Cool completely. Leaving the leather on the parchment, cut the leather into ribbons. Roll and store in an airtight container for up to 1 week.

Watermelon

A picnic and a playful summer afternoon at our neighborhood park never seems to get old (at least not yet). It's those simple summer pleasures that create great memories. But during those long summer days, like a predictable TV sitcom, the local ice-cream truck always seems to roll by just when a late-afternoon game of chase has left my kids tired, parched, and hungry. It's as if the truck driver navigates with a fine-tuned radar—his timing is uncanny.

I've overheard many a mom say that she forgot her purse to dodge the bullet. Instead, I employ this strategy: the Sweet Alternative. When the truck arrives, we head home to make our own pops. The kids experiment and create their own concoctions—tart ones with lemon and lime, sweet ones with berries, honey, and yogurt, and still more with any kind of melon they can find. Scooping melon into adorable little balls is delicious fun!

Watermelon is one of those irresistibly refreshing melons. It's a summertime staple in our house (for good reason). Thirst quenching (it's 92 percent water) and packed with lycopene,[4] watermelon is a healthy way to beat the heat. It's fun to scoop, fun to blend into a treat, and even more fun to eat with its sweet juice running down your chin. Better than anything the ice-cream truck can offer!

Make It a Game: 5 points
Eat Your Colors: Red, Yellow/Orange

Invite Exploration

"What is an easy way to scoop the flesh out of a watermelon?"

"After you're done scooping out the watermelon, what is an easy way to get the remaining juice out of the melon?"

Watermelon-Lime Ice Pops

There's no better way to cool rising temperatures than with a homemade frosty treat. Watermelon-Lime Ice Pops to the rescue! This recipe is colorful, easy, and tasty. With perfectly ripe summer fruit, we didn't need a drop of sugar to sweeten this treat. A welcome change from the frozen treats that come from a box—and at a fraction of the cost.

PREP TIME: 10 minutes

Wait time: 20 to 60 minutes

Makes about 9 ice pops

INGREDIENTS:

4 cups seedless watermelon balls

3 fresh limes

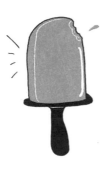

DIRECTIONS:

1 Place the watermelon in a food processor and process until smooth. Wrap a kitchen towel around the rim of the food processor to keep the juice from flowing out.

2 Run the watermelon puree through a sieve or food mill into a bowl.

3 Using a citrus press, squeeze the juice from the limes into the bowl with the watermelon puree and stir gently to combine.

4 Pour the juice into ice pop molds and freeze for about an hour.

Tip For faster pops, we use a Zoku ice pop maker. For best results when using a Zoku, chill the watermelon-lime juice for about 10 minutes before loading it into the Popsicle maker.

Cook Together

Beginners: Scoop the watermelon. Squeeze the lime juice. Run the food processor. Fill the Popsicle molds.

Tip: You can cut the watermelon with a knife, but my kids think the melon baller is much more fun, and it makes it easier for them to work independently.

Watermelon Gazpacho

Juicy, thirst-quenching watermelon paired with garden-fresh cherry tomatoes come together to create this refreshing variation on a classic Spanish summer soup. Encourage tasters by serving this chilled soup in eggcups, garnished with mini celery sticks.

PREP TIME: 15 minutes

WAIT TIME: 60 minutes

Serves 4

INGREDIENTS:

4 cups watermelon balls

1 cup chopped cherry tomatoes

½ cup diced celery, plus more for garnish

2 tablespoons fresh lime juice (from 1 lime)

2 tablespoons extra-virgin olive oil

Kosher salt and freshly ground black pepper

DIRECTIONS:

1 In the bowl of a food processor, combine the watermelon, tomatoes, celery, lime juice, and oil. Process for 2 minutes, or until the mixture is smooth and the texture is uniform.

2 Season with salt and pepper to taste.

3 Transfer to a large bowl and chill for 1 hour.

4 Serve in small cups, garnished with celery sticks or a few celery leaves.

Buy in Season Watermelons are supposed to be easy to grow, but despite our best gardening efforts, the melons in our kitchen garden didn't make it. Instead, we sourced our sweet summer giant from the local farmers' market—the next best thing to your garden and a fun way to let your kids discover what's in season.

Watermelon Smoothie

Beat the late-afternoon summer heat with a refreshing smoothie packed with goodness. When preparing a watermelon, place a few cups of the cut fruit on a baking sheet and freeze. Use your watermelon cubes in your smoothie for an extra blast of coolness.

PREP TIME: 10 minutes

COOK TIME: 0 minutes

Serves 4

INGREDIENTS:

2 cups seedless watermelon balls

1 cup chopped strawberries

2 tablespoons fresh lime juice (from 1 lime)

1 tablespoon honey

DIRECTIONS:

1 In a blender, combine the watermelon, strawberries, lime juice, and honey. Blend on high speed for 2 minutes, or until the ingredients are fully combined.

Tip *If you're using frozen watermelon cubes, add ½ cup water or fresh-squeezed orange juice to make it easier to blend.*

Keep Trying Experiment with combining watermelon with other foods growing in your garden. Tomato, cucumber, mint, and thyme are great places to start.

Lavender

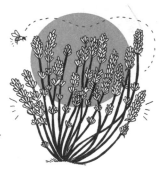

The notion of eating a flower is wonderfully intriguing to my kids. They've grown to recognize that we can eat many parts of a plant—leaves (like kale) or roots (like carrots) or fruit (like lemons) or seeds (like pumpkin)—but eating a flower evokes an entirely different feeling. For my kids, it's the garden equivalent of the intricate rosettes lining a birthday cake.

Although there are many types of edible flowers, the one I like best is lavender. True, it can be overpowering if steeped too long or if you use the wrong variety, but traditional English lavender used gently can be a wonderful sidekick in summer sweets. Its distinct aroma lingers on little fingers, and when brewed, it fills up the whole house with its welcoming scent. The other reason I love lavender is that it's super easy to grow. It needs only three conditions: sunshine, lack of water, and frequent harvesting. The perfect combination for a busy family with a mom who is prone to forget watering! Give your starter plants a home in a sunny, well-drained location, and they will reward you with buds all summer long.

When summer fever takes over, and that edgy "I'm bored" feeling starts to permeate the house, send the kids out to pick lavender and, like magic, calm will be restored. Whether it's aromatherapy working its wonders, or just the peace that comes with a simple, outdoor activity, lavender has many benefits to offer.

Make It a Game: 15 points
Eat Your Colors: Blue/Purple

Invite Exploration

"I wonder why some flowers are edible and others are not? How can you tell the difference?"

Lavender Lemonade

Infusing lavender into fresh lemonade adds a flavorful twist to this classic summer sipper and takes lemonade stand sales to new heights! Picking the buds is great fun for kids, but be sure to work over a rimmed baking sheet so those little jewels don't end up all over your house like glitter. Steeping lavender creates a tea that can be enjoyed on its own or infused into other recipes, from lemonade to cakes and cookies.

PREP TIME: 10 minutes

Cook time: 10 minutes

Serves 6

INGREDIENTS:

½ cup fresh English lavender

4 lemons

½ cup honey

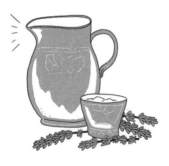

DIRECTIONS:

1 Harvest a large handful of lavender. Working over a rimmed baking sheet, remove the buds from the stems and place them in a measuring cup. Set aside.

2 Using a citrus press, squeeze the juice from the lemons into a small bowl. Set aside.

3 In a small pot, bring 5½ cups water to a boil. Reduce the heat to maintain a simmer, add the lavender buds, then cover and simmer for 10 minutes.

4 Line a colander with a paper towel, then strain the lavender water through the paper towel into a large bowl. Press gently on the lavender to extract all of its oils. Transfer the water to a pitcher.

Cook Together

Beginners: Harvest the lavender. Remove the buds. Squeeze the lemons. Stir the lemonade.

Tip: When your kids are working with lavender, use a rimmed baking sheet. When James removes buds from sprigs of lavender, escapees fly everywhere. A rimmed baking sheet easily captures any rogue buds and gives me the comfort to let him work on his own without making a huge mess. At the end, corral the buds from the rimmed baking sheet into your bowl.

5 Stir the honey into the warm lavender water until dissolved.

6 Once cooled, add the lemon juice and a handful of ice to the honey-lavender mixture and stir gently.

7 Serve cold.

> **Grow It** The best lavender for cooking is the English variety. Plant in a sunny location. Soil should drain well and be on the dry side. You don't need to water lavender all that frequently. We found it easiest to start our lavender from small plants as opposed to seeds.

Lavender Mint Tea

As a little girl, I loved a tea party. I've spent years collecting teacups of every shape and color—each one has a story. Instead of locking them up for special occasions, I use them regularly with my kids. They rummage through the cabinet to find their treasure—often a mismatched set—and together we enjoy tea with herbs from our garden (or hot cocoa, depending on the season). It's another fun way to gather around the table and make memories. This tea is a summertime favorite.

PREP TIME: 5 minutes
COOK TIME: 10 to 15 minutes
Serves 4

INGREDIENTS:
1 teaspoon fresh English lavender buds
5 fresh mint leaves
Lemon

DIRECTIONS:

1 In a small saucepan, bring 2 cups water to a boil.

2 Place the lavender buds and mint leaves in the metal basket of your teapot or loose tea infuser. To release more oils, gently crush the leaves in your hand first.

3 Add the water and steep the herbs in your teapot for 10 to 15 minutes, depending on how strong you and your kids prefer the taste.

4 Add a squeeze of lemon before serving, if you like.

Flaxseeds

As with so many things in life, big things come in small packages. In this case, the small package is a seed, and the big thing it delivers is a daily dose of omega-3s—the same powerful fats that make fish nutritious (though in a slightly different form). A boost of fiber gives its nutritional punch additional power. The beauty of this tiny package is the ease with which we can work it into almost all of our favorite foods, effortlessly giving them an extra boost. Flaxseeds are the food equivalent to Tinker Bell's pixie dust—just a sprinkle delivers remarkable results.

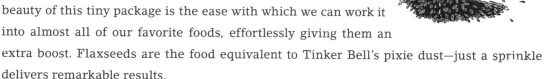

Most nutritionists recommend grinding flaxseeds, to make them easier to digest.[5] Although my kids would have gone to town with a mortar and pestle had I given them the chance, I found it much more convenient to just pick up a bag of ground flaxseeds from the store and get cooking. The easiest way to "cook" with flaxseeds is to simply sprinkle it on your oatmeal or yogurt or blend it into a smoothie and call it a day. But you can also work it into your baking, which is where my kids had the most fun experimenting. First, we decided to make a healthier version of their favorite packaged granola bar. Then we started adding flaxseed meal to our other favorite recipes like Zucchini Muffins (page 183), Mini Pear-Apple Crisp (page 106), and Strawberry-Rhubarb Crisp (page 218), to delicious results.

When you're cooking with your kids, encourage them to experiment with adding this beneficial ingredient to your dishes. Pick the low-hanging fruit first, like smoothies, but also encourage them to branch out and try this simple ingredient in a new way. They may come up with something clever and tasty.

> ### Invite Exploration
> "Which of our favorite family recipes could benefit from a boost of flaxseeds?"

Make It a Game: 10 points
Eat Your Colors: Protein

Power Bars

This homemade granola bar recipe gets its power from flaxseeds. It is fun to make together and can easily be modified to feature your favorite fixings. These bars are crunchy and crumbly. When you're done cutting them, the baking sheet will be filled with tasty chunks of granola—perfect for sprinkling over yogurt parfaits.

PREP TIME: 10 minutes
COOK TIME: 35 minutes
Makes 16 bars

INGREDIENTS:

4 cups old-fashioned rolled oats

¼ cup flaxseed meal

¼ cup whole wheat all-purpose flour

½ cup unsweetened shredded coconut

½ teaspoon ground cinnamon

½ teaspoon kosher salt

½ cup grapeseed oil

½ cup honey

¼ cup maple syrup

1 cup dark chocolate chips or dried cranberries

DIRECTIONS:

1 Preheat the oven to 325°F. Line a 9 x 9-inch baking pan with parchment paper.

2 In a large bowl, combine the oats, flax meal, flour, coconut, cinnamon, and salt.

3 Add the oil, honey, and maple syrup to the dry mixture. Stir to combine.

4 Add the chocolate chips and mix well.

5 Let your kids press the granola mixture firmly into the prepared pan. Put a little oil on your hands to prevent the granola from sticking to your fingers.

6 Bake for 35 minutes, or until golden brown. The mixture will still be soft to the touch when you take it out of the oven.

7 Cool, then cut into bars.

Tip Add the oil, then the honey, using the same measuring cup. The oil will make it easy for the honey to slip right off into the bowl.

Tip This is another great recipe to let your kids come up with their own mix of ingredients. Encourage them to experiment with different flavor combinations.

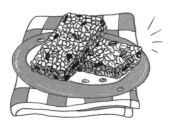

Cook Together

Beginners: Combine the ingredients. Press the mixture into the pan.

Keep Trying We tried several granola recipes before landing on one that we liked. Some of our recipes were too crumbly, others too chewy. You may have a similar experience as your kids try new ingredients in their mix. Instead of getting frustrated, view it as an opportunity to experiment.

Do the Math How much do you spend on the packaged organic granola bars that regularly appear in your kids' lunchboxes? Conservatively, in our house, it was about $100 per child per year. Then stop and look at the ingredients list. It's less healthy than you think. "Convenience!" you reply, and I completely understand. As a busy parent, I need a grab-and-go solution some mornings, too. But when I created this simple recipe for homemade granola bars, I was surprised at how easy, tasty, and simple it is to make your own granola bars at home for a fraction of the cost.

Strawberry-Banana Smoothie

A quick-and-easy way to work flaxseeds—and their healthy oils—into your diet is to blend them into a smoothie. Made with Greek yogurt, this sipper gives your kids an extra boost of protein, too.

PREP TIME: 5 minutes

COOK TIME: 0 minutes

Serves 4

INGREDIENTS:

1 large banana

1 cup frozen strawberries

½ cup nonfat plain Greek yogurt

½ cup nonfat milk

1 tablespoon flaxseed meal

DIRECTIONS:

1 In a blender, combine the banana, strawberries, yogurt, milk, and flaxseed meal. Blend for 1 to 2 minutes, or until the mixture is thoroughly combined and no large chunks of fruit remain.

Tip Store seeds and nuts in the freezer or refrigerator. Keeping them cold retains their healthy oils, which will oxidize if they are kept at room temperature.

Cook Together

Invite your kids to add 1 tablespoon of maple syrup or honey for a touch of extra sweetness.

Chickpeas

Who doesn't love a dip? Like a summer campfire, everyone seems to gather around them when they appear and happiness ensues. For Catherine and James, the chance to dip their veggies simply makes food more fun.

Which brings me to chickpeas.

These pea-size beans pack a punch. Chock-full of plant protein, chickpeas are a great source of fiber and nutrients, including iron and zinc.[6] Homemade hummus made with chickpeas is the most versatile base I've found for creating colorful, healthy dips. The basic version, with roasted garlic and lemon, is easy to make; saves well; and can be used as a dip, spread, or condiment with equal success. Beyond the basics, chickpeas can be blended with sweet peas, edamame, or peppers to make a colorful array of dips. Create a color wheel and dip your colors in your colors!

Dips aren't the only way this lovely legume can help you. Roast them in a low oven, like edamame beans, and you've got a perfect after-school snack. Or sauté them with your favorite spices and stir in a hearty leafy green, like kale, for a quick-and-easy main. Their ease can't be beat, and on a busy mom's schedule, that earns them extra points.

Make It a Game: 10 points
Eat Your Colors: Protein

Invite Exploration

"What other veggies could we blend into our hummus?"

Healthy Homemade Hummus

This easy dip can be made fast or slow. For maximum flavor, go slow. Toast sesame seeds to make your own tahini and soak dried chickpeas overnight. For a quick hit, use canned chickpeas and store-bought tahini (just look for one with ingredients you can identify). This homemade hummus outshines any store-bought hummus by a long shot. From a taste perspective, there is no comparison. Make this dip on the weekend and enjoy with a variety of dishes all week.

PREP TIME: 10 minutes

Cook time: 0 minutes

Makes about 2 cups

INGREDIENTS:

2 cups chickpeas, drained and rinsed

½ cup extra-virgin olive oil, plus more for drizzling

1 teaspoon tahini, store-bought or fresh (see page 279)

2 tablespoons fresh lemon juice (from 1 lemon)

1 large clove Roasted Garlic (page 69)

½ teaspoon kosher salt

Sweet paprika, for sprinkling

Fresh-cut veggies and fruit, for serving

DIRECTIONS:

1 In the bowl of a food processor, combine the chickpeas, oil, tahini, lemon juice, roasted garlic, and salt. Process until smooth, about 2 minutes. Add a touch more olive oil to adjust the consistency, if you like.

2 Chill for 15 minutes.

3 Serve cold, with a drizzle of olive oil and a sprinkle of paprika alongside fresh-cut veggies like peppers, cauliflower, broccoli, and cucumber, as well as crunchy fruits like apples.

Tip *I prefer to use dried chickpeas for better flavor. If you choose this route, plan ahead. In a large bowl, add the dried chickpeas and cover fully with water. Soak overnight. Drain, then boil gently for about an hour and a half. Let cool before using. If you choose to use chickpeas from a can, be sure to pick a brand that is BPA-free.*

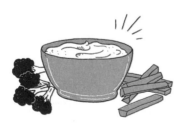

Cook Together

Beginners: Measure and load the ingredients. Run the food processor.

Experts: Cut the vegetables.

Sweet Pea Hummus

Follow the directions for Healthy Homemade Hummus, substituting 1 cup fresh shelled sweet peas (from about 1 pound of peas in the pod) for 1 cup of the chickpeas.

Roasted Red Pepper Hummus

Follow the directions for Healthy Homemade Hummus, substituting 1 cup roasted red peppers for 1 cup of the chickpeas.

Homemade Tahini

In a large sauté pan, lightly toast 1 cup sesame seeds over medium heat until golden brown and fragrant, about 2 minutes. Let cool. In a food processor, combine the toasted seeds with ⅓ cup extra-virgin olive oil and process until smooth, 2 to 3 minutes. Store in a glass container in the refrigerator for up to 1 week. Use the tahini to make hummus or add it to tamari to make a sauce for chicken or beef.

Roasted Chickpea Pop'ems

Follow the directions for Roasted Edamame Pop'ems (page 142), substituting 2 cups chickpeas for the edamame. Let your kids experiment with different seasonings, like kosher salt, garlic salt, cumin, and paprika.

Hearty Chickpea Curry

As your kids warm to the flavor and texture of chickpeas, you can start working them into main dishes like this hearty stew. Catherine loves the soulful flavor of chicken curry, so we've started experimenting with this variation made with chickpeas. It's quick and easy, which makes it perfect for a busy weeknight. Use spinach or kale, whichever leafy green you and your kids prefer.

PREP TIME: 5 minutes

COOK TIME: 7 minutes

Serves 4

INGREDIENTS:

1½ cups chickpeas

3 tablespoons grapeseed oil

¼ cup chopped red onion (about ¼ medium onion)

1 tablespoon finely chopped peeled fresh ginger

1 tablespoon ground cumin

2 cups spinach

1½ cups chopped tomatoes

1 teaspoon kosher salt

¼ cup nonfat plain Greek yogurt

Cooked brown rice, for serving

DIRECTIONS:

1   Drain and rinse the chickpeas. Set aside.

2   Heat a large sauté pan over medium-high heat. Add the oil, onion, ginger, and cumin and cook for 2 minutes, or until the onions have softened.

3   Add the chickpeas, spinach, tomatoes, and salt. Stir to combine. Cook for 4 to 5 minutes, or until the spinach has wilted and the mixture is bubbling.

4   Remove from the heat. Stir in the yogurt.

5   Serve over brown rice

Workhorse Recipes

INSTEAD OF GETTING FANCY, IT'S BEST TO PREPARE A MAIN DISH THAT YOU KNOW YOUR KIDS will love and pair it with a combination of colorful foods (some familiar, some new) to round out your meals. There are a few main dishes that I serve each week. They vary slightly by season, but for the most part these recipes stay pretty true to form so that I can count on them to do the job each night.

Chicken

Easy Roasted Chicken (*page 282*)

Simple Sautéed Chicken (*page 283*)

Beef

Tasty Beef Skewers (*page 284*)

Anthony's Famous Short Ribs (*page 285*)

Pork

Gigi's Roasted Pork Tenderloin (*page 286*)

Fish

Ginger-Soy Glazed Cod (*page 287*)

Tofu

Pan-Seared Tofu Slices (*page 288*)

Easy Roasted Chicken

A simple roasted chicken is my go-to main dish on busy weeknights. Once you get the hang of it, you'll find it's easier than you think to make roast chicken at home, and the taste is so much better than the dry rotisserie chickens sitting on the shelf at your local grocery store. Those may be convenient, but they definitely don't win on flavor. I always save some extras to work into meals throughout the week.

PREP TIME: 10 minutes

COOK TIME: 60 minutes

SERVES 4

INGREDIENTS:

1 (1½-pound) whole chicken

Garlic powder

Kosher salt and freshly ground black pepper

A few sprigs fresh rosemary or thyme

DIRECTIONS:

1 Preheat the oven to 400°F.

2 Trim the chicken and place in a large cast-iron roasting pan. Season with garlic powder, salt, and pepper. Stuff the cavity with a handful of fresh herbs from your garden. Our favorites are rosemary or thyme.

3 Roast for 60 minutes, or until the skin is crispy and the meat is cooked through. It's that easy, really.

Tip *Cover with aluminum foil if the chicken starts to smoke or brown too much.*

Simple Sautéed Chicken

This recipe is an easy substitute for breaded chicken Parmesan. The delicious sauce is what my kids love most. I love that it takes only ten minutes to make!

PREP TIME: 5 minutes

COOK TIME: 10 minutes

SERVES 4

INGREDIENTS:

½ teaspoon garlic powder

½ teaspoon kosher salt

1½ pounds boneless chicken thigh pieces, trimmed of fat

1 tablespoon extra-virgin olive oil

¼ cup white wine or lemon juice

1 tablespoon unsalted butter

DIRECTIONS:

1 In a small bowl, combine the garlic powder and salt. Season both sides of the chicken pieces with the garlic powder mixture.

2 Heat a large sauté pan over medium heat. Add the oil, then the chicken pieces. Cook for 5 to 7 minutes, or until the pan side of the chicken is browned.

3 Flip the chicken pieces and cook for 5 to 7 minutes more, or until the chicken is cooked through and bounces back when pressed with a fork. Transfer the chicken to a plate and set aside.

4 Deglaze the pan with the white wine and butter, scraping up the browned bits from the bottom of the pan with a wooden spoon. Reduce the heat and simmer for 2 to 3 minutes, or until the mixture has reduced slightly.

5 Drizzle the sauce over the chicken before serving.

Thanks to Amy Fothergill, the Family Chef, for teaching me this simple and tasty recipe.

Tasty Beef Skewers

The combination of peanut butter and tamari makes the flavor of these beef skewers outstanding. For maximum impact, make the beef a day ahead and let it marinate in the refrigerator.

PREP TIME: 10 minutes

COOK TIME: 10 to 12 minutes

SERVES 4

INGREDIENTS:

2 tablespoons peanut butter

2 tablespoons tamari

1 tablespoon mirin

1 clove garlic, finely chopped

1 tablespoon light brown sugar

1 pound flank steak, cut into ½-inch cubes

DIRECTIONS:

1 Preheat the oven to 400°F. Line a rimmed baking sheet with foil. Place 12 wooden skewers in a large cup of water to soak.

2 In a large bowl, combine the peanut butter, tamari, mirin, garlic, and sugar. Stir until the mixture forms a paste.

3 Add the beef and stir gently to thoroughly coat the meat.

4 Arrange a few pieces of beef on each skewer. Set the skewers on the lined baking sheet.

5 Bake for 10 to 12 minutes, or until the meat is cooked but still pink in the center.

6 Serve immediately.

Tip *You can skip the skewers and just cook the beef directly on the lined baking sheet, if you prefer. The skewers make it more fun, though!*

Anthony's Famous Short Ribs

This recipe takes an investment in time. But what this dish lacks in speed it makes up for (many times over) in taste. It is one of our all-time favorite main dishes. Make it over the weekend, and I promise, you will be rewarded all week long.

PREP TIME: 15 minutes

COOK TIME: 2 hours, 35 minutes

SERVES 8

INGREDIENTS:

5 pounds English-cut short ribs

Kosher salt and freshly ground black pepper

1 large onion, coarsely chopped

6 cloves garlic, coarsely chopped

6 large carrots, cut into 1-inch pieces

6 large stalks celery, cut into 1-inch pieces

2 tablespoons whole wheat all-purpose flour

2 cups red wine

Chicken Broth (page 99)

1 bay leaf

2 cinnamon sticks

DIRECTIONS:

1   Preheat the oven to 450°F.

2   Liberally season the ribs with salt and pepper. Place the meat bone-side down in a large roasting pan, cover with aluminum foil, and roast for 15 minutes. Turn the meat, then roast for 15 minutes more, or until the meat is crispy on the edges.

3   Remove the ribs and reduce the oven temperature to 250°F. Set the roasted meat aside on a plate lined with paper towels. Discard the oil, leaving just enough in the pan to sauté the vegetables.

4   Heat the roasting pan over medium heat on your stovetop over two burners. Sauté the onion for 2 minutes, or until it begins to turn brown and soften. Add the garlic, carrots, and celery and sauté for 3 minutes more, or until the veggies brown on the edges.

5   Add the flour to the veggies and stir to combine. Then add the wine and scrape up the remaining bits of meat from the bottom of the pan.

6   Transfer the ribs to a large, ovenproof pot and pour the veggie mixture over the meat. Add enough broth to cover the ribs, then add the bay leaf and cinnamon sticks.

7   Cover the pot and bake for 2 hours, or until the meat falls off the bone.

8   Remove the ribs and place in a large serving dish. Discard the cooked vegetables. Use the remaining liquid as your gravy.

Tip *You can also make this recipe in a slow cooker set to low for 6 hours.*

Gigi's Roasted Pork Tenderloin

I learned this simple recipe from my mom. It's perfect for a weeknight because it's quick, easy, and delicious. You don't have to tie the meat, but if you do, the slices will be more round and good-looking when you slice them. I like to serve this dish with Easy Asian Pear Sauce (page 165), Asian Plum Sauce (page 212), or applesauce.

PREP TIME: 10 minutes

COOK TIME: 20 minutes

SERVES 4

INGREDIENTS:

1 pound pork tenderloin

1 tablespoon extra-virgin olive oil

1 tablespoon tamari or soy sauce

Kosher salt and freshly ground black pepper

DIRECTIONS:

1   Preheat the oven to 475°F. Line a large roasting pan with foil or parchment paper.

2   Tie the tenderloin with twine at even intervals, spaced about 2 inches apart.

3   In a small bowl, combine the oil and tamari. Using a pastry brush, paint the meat with the dressing. Season with salt and pepper.

4   Place the meat in the roasting pan and cook for 20 minutes, or until the meat is crispy on the edges but pink in the center. If the roast is too pink in the center, cover with foil and let rest on a cutting board for 10 minutes. It's best not to overcook the meat, or it will be dry and tough.

Tip *Sear the meat before cooking for an extra-crispy crust.*

Ginger-Soy Glazed Cod

This dish has just enough flavor to win over picky palates. Wrapping the fish in aluminum foil or parchment paper and baking it in the oven allows the fish to steam beautifully and saves you time to prep your sides.

PREP TIME: 10 minutes

COOK TIME: 10 minutes

SERVES 4

INGREDIENTS:

1 pound fresh cod fillet

3 tablespoons tamari or soy sauce

1 tablespoon finely chopped peeled fresh ginger

1 tablespoon honey

DIRECTIONS:

1 Preheat the oven to 350°F.

2 Rinse the fish and place it on a large piece of foil or parchment paper on a rimmed baking sheet. Turn up the edges of the foil to create a barrier for your marinade.

3 In a small bowl, whisk together the tamari, ginger, and honey.

4 Pour the ginger dressing over the fish. Fold up the edges of the foil around the fish and seal to create a packet.

5 Bake for 10 minutes, or until the fish is flaky and cooked through.

Tip *Garnish with chopped green onions.*

Pan-Seared Tofu Slices

This recipe boasts big flavor but no meat. It's great for your meatless dinner night. But it's so quick and easy that you may find that you reach for this recipe more than once a week.

PREP TIME: 10 minutes

COOK TIME: 10 minutes

SERVES 4

INGREDIENTS:

1 pound extra-firm tofu

2 tablespoons nori flakes

1 teaspoon sesame seeds

4 tablespoons grapeseed oil

DIRECTIONS:

1 Place the block of tofu on a plate lined with paper towels. Cover the tofu with more paper towels and press gently to remove the water.

2 Slice the tofu into ½-inch squares. Set aside.

3 In a small baking dish, combine the nori flakes and sesame seeds. Roll the edges of each tofu square in the nori mixture.

4 Heat a large sauté pan over medium heat. Add half the oil, then half of the tofu squares. Cook for 3 minutes, or until the tofu is crispy on the bottom. Flip and cook for 3 minutes more, until golden brown. Repeat for the remaining tofu, refreshing the oil between batches.

5 Serve immediately.

Tip *Press the tofu gently, or it will crumble and make a mess in the pan.*

APPENDIX B

Points Chart

THE SAMPLE MENU BELOW GIVES AN EXAMPLE OF HOW TO calculate your score. In this meal, kale, carrots, and strawberries make up the three colors—green, yellow/orange, and red. Protein points are earned by eating a serving of roasted chicken, healthy grains points from brown rice, and liquid points from a glass of water. Bonus points are awarded for trying a new food—kale—even if your child simply puts it in his mouth and spits it out.

> Main: Roasted chicken (10 protein points)
> New Food: Kale (15 green points PLUS 2x all of your
> points for this meal)
> Side: Carrots (10 yellow/orange points)
> Healthy Grains: Brown rice (5 healthy grains points)
> Drink: Water (5 liquid points)
> Dessert: Strawberries (5 red points)

> Total: 50 points x 2 for trying a new food = 100 points

Record your score only if your plate meets these requirements, and your kids actually eat it. For some families, it's helpful to set a points target for the week.

Formula for a Winning Plate

3 colors + 1 protein + 1 healthy grain + 1 liquid = 30 points

The more points the better.

No maximum points for colors. Earn as many as you like.

Limit protein and healthy grains points to one serving at each meal.

Double all of the points on your plate for trying a new food.

Award points for water and milk, but not juice or soda.

The 52 New Foods Challenge Points Chart

Points	Green	Yellow / Orange	Blue / Purple	Red	White
5	**Apples**, Grapes, Honeydew, Kiwi, Lemons, Limes, **Pears**	**Apples**, Apricots, **Asian pears**, Bananas, Cantaloupe, **Grapefruit**, **Kumquats**, Lemon, Mangoes, Nectarines, **Oranges**, **Peaches**, **Pears**, **Persimmons**, Pineapples, Tangerines	**Blackberries**, **Black currants**, Blueberries, Dates, Elderberries, Figs, Grapes, **Lavender**, **Plums**, Prunes, Purple potatoes	**Apples**, Blood oranges, **Cherries**, Cranberries, **Grapefruit**, Guava, Papaya, Pears, **Pomegranate**, Potatoes, Raspberries, **Strawberries**, **Watermelon**	Nectarines, **Peaches**, Potatoes
10	**Avocados**, **Broccoflower (Romanesco)**, Broccoli, Celery, **Cucumbers**, **Edamame**, **Green beans**, Green bell peppers, Olives, **Peas**, Tomatillos, **Zucchini**	Carrots, **Corn**, Summer squash, **Tomatoes**, Yellow bell peppers	Olives, **Cauliflower**, Purple corn, Purple bell peppers	**Rainbow carrots**, Red bell peppers, **Tomatoes**	**Cauliflower**, **Corn**, **Mushrooms**
15	**Artichokes**, Arugula, **Asparagus**, **Basil**, **Bok choy**, **Brussels sprouts**, **Butter Lettuce**, Cabbage, Chard, Endive, **Kale**, **Okra**, **Onions**, Pea shoots, **Romanesco**, Seaweed, Spinach	Beets, **Butternut squash**, **Pumpkin**, **Sweet potatoes**	Black salsify, **Eggplant**, Purple asparagus, Purple cabbage, Purple endive, **Radicchio**	Beets, Chili peppers, **Radishes**, Rainbow Chard, Red Onions, **Rhubarb**, Rutabaga	Celery root, Fennel, **Garlic**, Ginger, Jícama, Kohlrabi, **Leeks**, **Onions**, Parsnips, Shallots, Turnips

Points	Proteins	Grains	Liquids
5		Brown rice, Couscous, **Flaxseed**, Oatmeal, Popcorn, **Quinoa**, **Whole wheat flour** (bread, tortillas, pasta)	Milk, Water
10	Almond butter, **Black beans**, Beef, **Chickpeas**, Cheese, Chicken, Eggs, **Fish**, Nuts, Peanut butter, **Sunflower butter**, Tofu, Yogurt		

Note: Foods highlighted in bold are part of the 52 New Foods Challenge.

Recipe Index by Type of Dish

Mains

Sides

Recipe Index by Ingredient

Acknowledgments

MANY WONDERFUL PEOPLE CAME TOGETHER TO BRING THIS BOOK TO LIFE. LIKE A FAMILY meal, *The 52 New Foods Challenge* was made special by what each person brought to the table.

My kind and wise friend Bill Draper encouraged me to journey down the path of writing this book and introduced me to Jim Levine, who believed in the seed of an idea. They were the catalysts for this adventure. I am deeply thankful for their support.

Danielle Svetcov—my extraordinary agent—orchestrated all of the pieces to make this project fly and keep it soaring. Without her immense talent none of this would have happened. Danielle's spirit and keen sense of direction helped me turn the seed I was nurturing into a story. She is equally my trusted adviser and friend.

The team at Avery/Gotham Books welcomed me into the Penguin Random House family with warm arms. I am grateful for their support and honored to be able to count myself as a "Penguin." Lucia Watson, my dedicated and talented editor, expertly guided this book through every stage of the editorial process with passion and confidence. From the start, she recognized the power of taking small steps to help families establish a lifetime of healthy habits—that this book isn't just about getting your kids to eat broccoli; it's about making your journey as a family more fulfilling, healthy, and fun. Lucia's sharp editorial eye helped me produce a book that is equally easy for busy parents as it is powerful in making healthy changes. I am deeply grateful for her support.

My heartfelt thanks to the entire time at Avery, including publishers Brian Tart and Bill Shinker, and the dedicated team of Lisa Johnson, Megan Newman, Farin Schlussel, Anne Kosmoski, Marisa Vigilante, Gabrielle Campo, and Claire Vaccaro for working tirelessly to bring it all together. It has been a pleasure working with such a talented team, and I appreciate everything that they did to make this book sing.

The illustrations in this book tell our story in another way, and this is where Summer Pierre's special gift shines through. Summer gave me another window into the world of food—I know you'll enjoy the view. My longtime friends at Classic Kids Photography, led by Megan Hird, captured the pictures for the cover. Megan has been taking pictures of my family since my babies were born. I am grateful that she shared her talent for this project.

Nationally renowned experts brought their skills to round out the story. Dr. Walter Willett, Dr. Christopher Gardner, Chef Ann Cooper, Frances Largeman-Roth, Raj Patel, Jesse Cool, Dr. Alan Greene, George Kembel, and Curt Ellis each helped broaden my understanding of the myriad issues that come together when making changes to a family's food environment. I am immensely thankful for their support and council. A special thanks goes to the team at Jamie Oliver's Food Revolution, especially Joanna Creed and Sarah Jane Gourlay. Jo and Sarah have been tremendous supporters of our family cooking adventures from the start. With their help, the 52 New Foods Challenge has inspired hundreds of thousands of families to have fun trying new foods each week.

Several families spent months testing recipes and reviewing the many iterations of this book. Thanks to Connie McArthur, Deirdre Horgan, Danielle Kling, Brenda Thompson, Cheri Myers, Erin Pasero, Katherine Lau, Kendra Peterson, Mei Chen, Nicole Taylor, Patricia Lee, Rebecca Wolfe, Roxanne Munson, Sarah Arron, Sophia Lee, Alexandra Olmsted, Jung Choi, Christina O'Neill, Verna Kuo, Reena Agarwal, Kim Laidlaw, Maria Gagliano, Kathie Heap, Jan Ellison Baszucki, Cristina Laureola, *and their families*, for carefully poring over every inch of this book and providing suggestions on what would make it even better. Special thanks to Ashley Pearson, who coordinated the countless copies of the manuscript that kept these readers reading!

Dedicated teachers inspired curiosity in my children and helped them develop the tools to express their ideas. Maya Sissoko helped Catherine find her voice that comes through in the poetry she wrote for this book. Heather Connolly, Emily Mitchell, Sam Modest, Pete Bowers, and Peter Koehler encouraged James to use his passion for patterns to inspire action in others. Carolee Fucigna taught us how to ask questions to inspire creative adventures together. Diane Rosenberg and Terry Lee generously provided access to our school garden for our many food adventures. I learned as much from these teachers as did my kids. I am incredibly thankful for their guidance.

My family has always stood by me—through all of my countless projects. I am grateful, *beyond measure*, for their unrelenting encouragement and love. Each person in my family played a special role—recipe testing and editing, reviewing and critiquing designs, helping me set up a special place off the beaten path to write this book, and fielding daily calls to celebrate the amazing moments and to provide support through the tough ones. My family filled me up with love and encouragement. I am incredibly thankful *to each and every one of them* for the gifts that they've given to me.

I plan to pay it forward.

My children, Catherine and James, are my inspiration. Each day, they show me the joy of seeing the world through new eyes. Their curiosity feeds my spirit. I love them with my whole heart. When I embarked on this adventure, I thought it was about teaching them. What I discovered was that, in fact, all the while they have been teaching me—and they are the *best* teachers anyone could have.

The person, above all people, to whom I owe heartfelt thanks is my husband, Anthony. This book isn't my book—it is our book. *The 52 New Foods Challenge* took the support of my whole family, and Anthony led the charge to make it happen. He gave me the unwavering support and encouragement that I needed to try something new. He believed in me, even when I didn't believe in myself. I am deeply grateful for everything that Anthony did to help me make this book a reality. He is the *best* partner any person could ask for, and I count my lucky stars that we're on this journey, together.

Citations

Start Your Challenge

1   McGonigal, Jane. *Reality Is Broken: Why Games Make Us Better and How They Can Change the World.* New York: Penguin, 2011.

2   Moss, Michael. *Salt Sugar Fat: How the Food Giants Hooked Us.* New York: Random House, 2013.

Eat Your Colors

1   Zampollo, Francesca, Kevin M. Kniffin, Brian Wansink, and Mitsuru Shimizu. "Food plating preferences of children: the importance of presentation on desire for diversity." *Acta Paediatrica* 101, no. 1 (2012): 61–6.

2   USDA. "Bisphenol A (BPA): Use in Food Contact Application." www.fda.gov/NewsEvents /PublicHealthFocus/ucmo64437.htm.

Cook Together

1   Vo, Lam Thuy. "What America Spends on Groceries." NPR, June 8, 2012, www.npr.org /blogs/money/2012/06/08/154568945/what-america-spends-on-groceries.

2   USDA Economic Research Service. "Food Expenditures [by Location (Home versus Away)]," Tables 2 and 3. www.ers.usda.gov/data-products/food-expenditures.aspx#.UcTPL -u9zz4.

3   Let's Move. "Learn the Facts," www.letsmove.gov/learn-facts/epidemic-childhood-obesity (accessed February 25, 2014).

Buy in Season

1   USDA. "What Are Added Sugars?" www.choosemyplate.gov/weight-management-calories/ calories/added-sugars.html (accessed March 2014).

2   USDA. "How Many Can I Have?" http://www.choosemyplate.gov/weight-management-calories/calories/empty-calories-amount.html (accessed May 19, 2014).

3   Harvard School of Public Health. "The Nutrition Source: Added Sugar in the Diet,"

http://www.hsph.harvard.edu/nutritionsource/carbohydrates/added-sugar-in-the-diet /(accessed March 2014).

4   David, Laurie. *The Family Cooks: 100+ Recipes to Get Your Family Craving Food That's Simple Tasty, and Incredibly Good for You.* New York: Rodale, 2014.

5   Environmental Working Group. "EWG's 2013 Shoppers' Guide to Pesticides in Produce." www.ewg.org/foodnews/summary.php.

Grow It

1   Gibbs, Lisa, Petra K. Staiger, Britt Johnson, et al. "Expanding children's food experiences: the impact of a school-based kitchen garden program." *Journal of Nutrition Education and Behavior* 45, no. 2 (2013): 137–46; Robinson-O'Brien, Ramona, Mary Story, and Stephanie Heim. "Impact of garden-based youth nutrition intervention programs: a review." *Journal of the American Dietetic Association* 109, no. 2 (2009): 273–80. McAleese, Jessica D., and Linda L. Rankin. "Garden-based nutrition education affects fruit and vegetable consumption in sixth-grade adolescents." *Journal of the American Dietetic Association* 107, no. 4 (2007): 662–665; Henry, Sarah. "Berkeley's New School Food Study: A Victory for Alice Waters," *The Atlantic*, September 23, 2010, www.theatlantic.com/health/archive/2010/09/ berkeleys-new-school-food-study-a-victory-for-alice-waters/63465.

2   Pollan, Michael. "Some of My Best Friends are Germs," *New York Times Magazine*, May 15, 2013, http://www.nytimes.com/2013/05/19/magazine/say-hello-to-the-100-trillion -bacteria-that-make-up-your-microbiome.html.

Keep Trying, Together

1   *The Oxford Handbook of Eating Disorders.* New York: Oxford University Press, 2010.

2   Greene Dr. Alan, interview with author.

3   Le Billon, Karen, *Getting to Yum: The 7 Secrets of Raising Eager Eaters.* New York: Harper-Collins, 2014.

4   Fisher, Jennifer O., Julie A. Mennella, Sheryl O. Hughes, et al. "Offering 'dip' promotes intake of a moderately-liked raw vegetable among preschoolers with genetic sensitivity to bitterness." *Journal of the Academy of Nutrition and Dietetics* 112, no. 2 (2012): 235–45.

Fall

1   USDA Food-a-Pedia, Sweet potato (yam), baked (no salt added), peel not eaten versus Potato, baked (no salt added), peel not eaten.

2   Harvard Health Publications. "Glycemic Index and Glycemic Load for 100+ Foods." www .health.harvard.edu/newsweek/Glycemic_index_and_glycemic_load_for_100_foods.htm.

3   Marsh, Bill. "Nutritional Weaklings in the Supermarket." *New York Times*, May 25, 2013, www.nytimes.com/interactive/2013/05/26/sunday-review/26corn-ch.html.

4   Cornell University Growing Guide. "Garlic," www.gardening.cornell.edu/homegardening /scene568b.html.

5   USDA. "Carrots with Character." www.ars.usda.gov/is/ar/archive/nov04/carrot1104.htm (accessed March 4, 2014).

6   Subramanian, Sushma. "Fact or Fiction: Raw Veggies are Healthier than Cooked Ones." *Scientific American*, March 31, 2009, www.scientificamerican.com/article/raw-veggies-are -healthier.

7   USDA Food-a-Pedia.

8   Volpe, Richard and Abigail Okrent. "Assessing the Healthfulness of Consumers' Grocery Purchases," *USDA,* November 2012, www.ers.usda.gov/publications/eib-economic -information-bulletin/eib102.aspx.

9   Nestle, Marion. "Whole Wheat Is Not the Whole Story." *Food Politics*, www.foodpolitics .com/2010/10/4087.

Winter

1   Madison, Deborah. *Vegetable Literacy: Cooking and Gardening with Twelve Families from the Edible Plant Kingdom*. Berkeley, CA: Ten Speed Press, 2013, 243–45.

2   Weil, Andrew. "Dr. Andrew Weil's Guide to Healthy Eating Part 2." p. 53.

3   USDA Food-a-Pedia.

Spring

1   USDA Food-a-Pedia.

2   Cornell University Growing Guide. "Peas," www.gardening.cornell.edu/homegardening /scene9697.html.

3   Largeman-Roth, Frances. *Eating in Color: Delicious, Healthy Recipes for You and Your Family*. New York: Stewart, Tabori & Chang, 2014.

4 Shulman, Martha Rose. "A Cherry Jubilee." *New York Times*, June 23, 2013, www.nytimes
   .com/2013/06/24/health/arugula-cherry-and-goat-cheese-salad.html.

5 Madison. *Vegetable Literacy*, 108–109.

6 Nestle, Marion. "The Mediterrean Diet: A Delicious Way to Prevent Heart Disease?"
   Food Politics, April 7, 2013, www.foodpolitics.com/2013/04/mediterranean-diet-what-it-is
   -benefits/.

7 USDA Food-a-Pedia.

Summer

1 Largeman-Roth. *Eating in Color*, 30.

2 USDA. "Adoption of Genetically Modified Crops in the U.S." 2012–2013, National Agricul-
   tural Statistics Service (NASS). Acreage. June 28, 2013. www.ers.usda.gov/data-products
   /adoption-of-genetically-engineered-crops-in-the-us.aspx.

3 Hirsheimer, Christopher and Peggy Knickerbocker. *The San Francisco Ferry Plaza Farmers' Market Cookbook: A Comprehensive Guide to Impeccable Produce.* San Francisco:
   Chronicle Books, 2006.

4 Largeman-Roth. *Eating in Color*, 25.

5 Parker-Pope, Tara. "How to Add Flaxseed to Your Diet." *New York Times*, June 3, 2011,
   well.blogs.nytimes.com/2011/06/03/how-to-add-flaxseed-to-your-diet.

6 USDA Food-a-Pedia.

7 USDA. "Bisphenol A (BPA).

Index